OCCUPATIONAL THERAPY AS A CAREER

An Introduction to the Field and a Structured Method for Observation

OCCUPATIONAL THERAPY AS A CAREER

An Introduction to the Field and a Structured Method for Observation

Laura L. Swanson Anderson, OTR/L
Fieldwork Coordinator
Occupational Therapy Program
St. Ambrose University
Davenport, Iowa

Christine K. Malaski, MS, OTR/L
Assistant Professor
Occupational Therapy Program
St. Ambrose University
Davenport, Iowa

F. A. DAVIS COMPANY • Philadelphia

F.A. Davis Company
1915 Arch Street
Philadelphia, PA 19103

Printed in the United States of America

Last digit indicates print number: 10 9 8 7 6 5 4 3 2 1

Publisher, Health Professions: Jean-François Vilain
Senior Editor: Lynn Borders Caldwell
Production Editor: Michael Schnee
Cover Designer: Alicia R. Baronsky

As new scientific information becomes available through basic and clinical research, recommended treatments and drug therapies undergo changes. The authors and publisher have done everything possible to make this book accurate, up to date, and in accord with accepted standards at the time of publication. The authors, editors, and publisher are not responsible for errors or omissions or for consequences from application of the book, and make no warranty, expressed or implied, with regard to the contents of the book. Any practice described in this book should be applied by the reader in accordance with professional standards of care used with regard to the unique circumstances that may apply in each situation. The reader is advised always to check product information (package inserts) for changes and new information regarding dose and contraindications before administering any drug. Caution is especially urged when using new or infrequently ordered drugs.

Library of Congress Cataloging-in-Publication Data

Anderson, Laura L. Swanson, 1969–
    Occupational therapy as a career : an introduction to the field
and a structured method for observation / Laura L. Swanson Anderson, Christine K. Malaski.
        p.   cm.
    Includes bibliographical references and index.
    ISBN 0-8036-0387-8 (alk. paper)
    1. Occupational therapy—Vocational guidance.   I. Malaski,   Christine K., 1965–   .   II. Title.
RM735.4.A53   1999
615.8'515'023—dc21

98-28653
CIP

Foreword

Deciding to enter occupational therapy (OT) can be a daunting task! Learning about the profession is exciting, confusing, challenging, and oftentimes frustrating. OT practitioners and educators recognize the important role they play in assisting individuals who are making this important career decision. For example, as Director of the Occupational Therapy Program at the University of Puget Sound, I rarely go a day without receiving a call from a preoccupational therapy student who asks numerous questions: "What is occupational therapy?" "Where do occupational therapists work?" "Is there a demand for occupational therapists?" "How do I go about observing different OT settings?" "What OT education programs are available?" Occupational therapy educators expect pre-OT students to begin to answer these questions on their own before they are accepted into an occupational therapy education program. To ensure that the OT applicant is making an informed career decision, most schools require applicants to complete extensive observation or volunteer hours in various OT settings.

When I first read Malaski's (1996) article "Giving Focus to Pre-OT,"* I immediately liked the idea of a handbook for pre-OT students to guide them through the "maze" of OT observations. With enthusiasm, I contacted the authors for more information. I soon learned that their handbook was a "work in progress" and the authors were thinking of refining it for publication. Now in final form, *Occupational Therapy as a Career* will serve as a valuable guide for students desiring to enter an occupational therapy education program. More than a handbook for observing OT, this text offers important basic information about the profession and how to proceed in exploring OT as a career. The information is concise, accurate, and organized in a way that directly answers the questions that pre-OT students ask most frequently.

Although *Occupational Therapy as a Career* is written explicitly for pre-OT students, OT supervisors working in various settings and other professionals who assist students in making career and educational decisions will find this text a handy resource. Clinicians, OT educators, career counselors, and admissions staff at higher-education institutions can refer to this book when responding to pre-OT student questions and guiding students toward meaningful observations and volunteer experiences in the field of occupational therapy. This text should be on the bookshelves of every occupational therapy program director and in the bookstores of the colleges and universities where those OT programs are offered.

---

*Malaski, C. (August 29, 1996). Giving focus to pre-OT. *OT Week, 10*(35). Bethesda, MD: American Occupational Therapy Association.

As students, clinicians, educators, and career guidance counselors discover and use this text, the task of learning (and helping others to learn) about occupational therapy should become less daunting. The authors of *Occupational Therapy as a Career* should be commended for writing such a practical and useful text. I know my prospective students will thank them. . . . I certainly do!

Katherine B. Stewart, MS, OTR, FAOTA
Clinical Associate Professor and Chair
Occupational Therapy Program
University of Puget Sound

Acknowledgments

The authors wish to acknowledge the following individuals for their contributions:

The numerous students whom we have guided through observation/volunteer experiences. It is our intent that this text will assist future students in the successful completion of observation/volunteer experiences and offer assistance in making effective career decisions. An article in *OT Week* led numerous clinicians and pre-OT students to request information about a previous version of this book; you helped this book become a reality!

Our supportive colleagues in the occupational therapy departments at St. Ambrose University and Cottage Hospital.

Nanette Miller and Marylainne Block
Reference Librarians

Lewis Sanborne
Academic Support, St. Ambrose University

Christopher Bradshaw and John Malaski for the illustrations.

Lynn Borders Caldwell for believing in this project and offering excellent assistance the entire way through.

The following individuals for reviewing the initial manuscript and the revisions that followed. Much gratitude and thanks is conveyed to them for their exceptional guidance and direction regarding the content of this book:

Marsha A. Chiumiento, COTA
Academic Fieldwork Coordinator
Occupational Therapy Assistant Program
Lasell College
Newton, Massachusetts

Nancy M. Klein, MS, OTR
Program Director/Assistant Professor
Occupational Therapy Assistant Program
St. Louis Community College—Meramec
St. Louis, Missouri

Kelvin Jerome Higgins, SFC/COTA
NCOIC OT Branch Class Advisory
Occupational Therapy Branch AHS
Fort Sam Houston
San Antonio, Texas

Katherine B. Stewart MS, OTR, FAOTA
Clinical Associate Professor and Chair
School of Occupational Therapy
University of Puget Sound
Tacoma, Washington

Jan Miller Polgar, PhD, BSCOT, MAOT
Assistant Professor
Occupational Therapy Program
University of Western Ontario
London, Ontario, Canada

Reg Urbanowski, OTR, MScOT
Associate Professor and Chair
Division of Occupational Therapy
School of Medicine
West Virginia University
Morgantown, West Virginia

Contents

Introduction and General Information 1

PART 2

Education   41

Observation Guidelines 53

Other Learning Activities 113

Conclusion 143

Appendices 147

Occupational Therapy is . . .

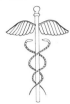

O

outcome oriented

C

caring professionals

C

creative

U

unique

P

purposeful activity use

A

activities of daily living

T

THERAPY

I

independence

O

organized

N

necessary

A

adaptable

L

leisure

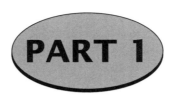

Introduction
and General
Information

1

How to Use This Book

On the pages that follow, specific instructions and guidelines are offered for the student, supervisor, and guidance counselor on how to use this book to maximize a student's experience in exploring and learning more about the profession of occupational therapy (OT).

For the Student Desiring to Enter Occupational Therapy School

This book was originally designed to help you learn all that you can during your required volunteer or observation hours at an OT clinic. It will help you become familiar with the many different practice areas in OT. Exploration of all of the practice areas presented in this book is not often a requirement for admission to OT school; the more familiar you are with them, however, the more prepared you will be to make effective career choices and to succeed in OT school.

This book is designed to be very flexible and adaptable. Depending on the length of your volunteer or observation experience, your supervisor may require you to complete certain assignments or the entire book. If your supervisor is not familiar with this book, please share it with him or her at the beginning of your volunteer or observation experience. What you complete within the book is up to you; the assignments and activities have been designed to guide your learning about the profession of OT. Completing assignments on your own demonstrates to your supervisor that you have initiative and motivation, as well as the ability to work independently.

Begin by reading through the first section of this book, "Introduction and General Information." Then complete the student preassessment ("Preobservation Assessment"). Share your answers with your supervisor so he or she may become familiar with your current knowledge level. Although you may be unable to answer all of the questions on the preassessment, your responses will assist you and your supervisor in developing and maximizing your learning experience. The results of your preassessment will let your supervisor know where you already have beginning knowledge and where you need to spend more time. Completing the preassessment may help you ask educated questions as well. Go over the "Observation Orientation

Documentation" and the "Observation Assignment List" with your supervisor to determine what is appropriate for that facility or clinic. Skim through the rest of the assignments and use any spare time you have to work on them. There may be "down time" during your observation or volunteer experience because of patient cancellations, therapist meetings, and time set aside to complete daily documentation. This down time may provide an excellent opportunity for you to share your work with your supervisor or other clinicians at the facility or clinic. Use your professional judgment and share your work with your supervisors at a convenient time for them.

The assignments to complete on your own are just that, but you may be able to use some of your spare time to complete them. Good time management is another important skill to show your supervisor, as well as other clinicians at the hospital or clinic. Maximize your time during your observation or volunteer experience. Do not sit and read magazines in the waiting room. You are in the clinic for a reason—to learn about OT! These assignments won't necessarily be shared with your volunteer sites, however.

Whenever you complete observation or volunteer time at a site, be sure to thank your supervisor. A good habit to develop is writing a short professional letter to your supervisors, thanking them for their time in assisting your learning and thanking the other clinicians who may have assisted you as well. Make certain to complete the "Release of Information Form" located in this book. You may ask your supervisor to write a reference for you now or in the future. Make certain that you and your supervisor have a signed copy of this form.

For the Supervisor

This book is designed to be as flexible as you need it to be. You may require your pre-OT students who call for observation hours to complete their hours more as volunteers (active and helping you as well as themselves) rather than just as passive observers. You may require them to follow a consistent schedule and to complete a certain number of hours (especially if you are often asked by students for a letter of reference to get into OT schools). Some students may come to you and already be following this book, or you can recommend it to them. You can follow this book exactly as it is written, or you can select what you believe will be most appropriate for your facility. The readings and assignments are simply suggestions and offer assignments for the students that will be of assistance to you and will help them make the most of their time.

Experience has taught many practicing clinicians that offering some structure to students provides for more efficient use of everyone's time. A little orientation time saves a lot of confusion. It should not require a great deal of your time to look over the assignments and they may help you guide the student. The "Supervisor's Evaluation of Observation Experience" may help you recall your thoughts about the particular student later on, when you may be asked to write a reference letter for the student applying to OT school. The students have been encouraged to use their time wisely and will have plenty to work on when your patient load is low or when you are busy with documentation and other tasks. A little time with students prior to their OT education will help them become better and more knowledgeable therapists later on.

For the Guidance Counselor, Occupational Therapy Program Director, and Admissions Counselor

This book is effective in a number of ways:

1. For students who are seriously considering a career in rehabilitation but are not certain whether OT is the career for them
2. For students who already know they wish to pursue a career in OT
3. For students who wish to gain more experience

For all of these reasons and more, this book is an excellent reference to assist the student in making career and educational decisions.

You may wish to keep copies of this book in stock in your bookstore for easy access by the students. Instructions are provided throughout the book for the student. Typically, it is up to the students to set up their observation or volunteer experience with an OT clinic. Depending on available facilities near your educational institution, you may recommend that a student start with an observation or volunteer experience at a general acute care hospital. Once the student has completed this experience, you may suggest or require, depending on your institution, that the student explore other OT practice areas. The book could also be required as part of your work-study program, possibly as an addition to the established Level I Fieldwork Experience. The text may be used as part of an Introduction to Occupational Therapy course. Instructions and explanations of each are provided. The book is conveniently divided into several categories to provide general information for students and assignments to help them make the most of their observation or volunteer experience.

For additional copies of this book, visit your local health science bookstore or contact the publisher:

F.A. Davis Company
1915 Arch Street
Philadelphia, PA 19103
Phone: 800-323-3555
E-mail: orders@fadavis.com
Web site: http://www.fadavis.com

Purpose of Readings and Assignments

The following provides an overview of what is covered in each chapter:

2 • **What Is Occupational Therapy?** Provides the student and guidance counselor with an overall basic understanding of the field of OT.

3 • **Health Professionals Related to Occupational Therapy:** Provides the student and guidance counselor with information on related health occupations and on how OT fits in with the interdisciplinary health-care team. Also helpful for students who are deciding whether OT or a related field would be the right career area for them.

4 • **What Is the Difference Between Occupational Therapy and Physical Therapy?** Assists the student and others in understanding what some of the differences are between OT and PT, since these two professions overlap in several areas.

5 • **How Do I Decide if Occupational Therapy Is the Right Career for Me?** Assists the potential OT student in deciding whether he or she has chosen the best career path.

6 • **Current Working Conditions Within the Profession of Occupational Therapy:** Provides information on job outlook, salary, other professionals who work with OTs, where OTs work, and training requirements.

7 • **Registered Occupational Therapist (OTR) and Certified Occupational Therapy Assistant (COTA) Role Delineation:** Provides the student with a basic explanation of the differences between OTR and COTA, as well as educational requirements for both.

8 • **How to Compare Occupational Therapy Schools:** Assists the student with his or her school selection process.

9 • **How to Apply to Occupational Therapy School:** Prepares the student for the application process and offers suggestions for making this process easier.

10 • **Pretest for Observation Experience:** Provides a test for pre-OT students to complete prior to their volunteer experience.

11 • **Professional Behavior Checklist:** Provides a checklist for self-assessment for the student and for others to provide the student with feedback. May be helpful in obtaining references for entering OT school.

12 • **Professional Feedback Forms:** Provides an opportunity for the pre-OT student to obtain feedback from those in the field.

13 • **Guidelines for Interaction with Patients:** Provides guidelines for the pre-OT student while he or she completes volunteer work.

14 • **Observation Assignment List:** Provides suggestions for students and supervisors to use while the student is completing volunteer hours. Allows for the observation time to be active learning rather than just passive observation. The supervisor at each site should determine with the student which assignments are most appropriate to complete.

15 • **Observation Orientation Documentation:** Provides a suggested orientation checklist to assist clinical supervisors in efficiently orienting pre-OT volunteers.

16 • **Confidentiality Statement:** A form for the student to sign at each clinical site to reinforce the importance of confidentiality.

17 • **Preobservation Assessment:** General questions, terms, and questions per-

taining to specific practice areas for the student to complete either before visiting a site or at the beginning of his or her volunteer experience. Helps the supervisor know the student's level of knowledge and helps the student know what questions to ask while completing volunteer time.

18 • **Professional Terminology Exercise:** Provides an introduction to terms used by physicians, nurses, and therapists.

19 • **Observation Worksheet for Practice Areas:** An opportunity for the supervising therapist to understand what the student knows about OT.

20 • **Observing a Therapist:** A worksheet for the student to complete on observations of different treatment sessions observed.

21 • **Patient Observation Tracking Sheet:** A suggested way for students to track the variety of patients they have observed.

22 • **Adaptive Equipment Scavenger Hunt:** Activity for student to complete while at the volunteer site to learn about adaptive equipment.

23 • **Time Management and Scheduling:** A place for the student to schedule his or her time in and out of the clinic.

24 • **Observer and Supervisor Weekly Report Form:** Structures feedback between the student and the clinical supervisor during a student's volunteer experience.

25 • **Release of Information Form:** Allows the supervisor to be used as a reference for the student who is applying to OT school, since information on students should be regarded with the same confidentiality as any patient or employee.

26 • **Supervisor's Evaluation of Observation Experience:** Provides written feedback for the pre-OT student upon completion of his or her volunteer experience; may assist the supervisor in recalling specifics on a student when asked to be a reference.

27 • **Observer's Evaluation of Experience:** Provides feedback to the clinical site on the student's experience.

28 • **Posttest of Observation Experience:** Tests pre-OT students on their basic knowledge of OT after their volunteer experience; students may compare it with the OT Quiz they completed prior to beginning their volunteer time.

29 • **Adaptive Equipment Matching Activity:** Helps students learn more about adaptive equipment commonly used.

30 • **Disability Experience Exercise:** For students to complete on their own time; a beginning exercise on empathy and an introduction to some OT theory.

31 • **Discussion of Occupational Therapy Assessment and Treatment of Simulated Disabilities:** Selected situations that might arise in the field.

32 • **Observation Experiences Without an OT:** Guides the student through self-study in the community.

33 • **Career Opportunity Assignment:** Encourages students to begin using the various OT publications and to start considering specific practice areas in which they are interested.

34 • **Goodbye and Good Luck!** A message just for the pre-OT student.
A • **Additional Resources:** Provides the student with basic information necessary to contact professional OT organizations.
B • **Answers for Quizzes:** Answers to the quizzes found throughout this book.
C • **High School Courses Helpful in Preparing for an Occupational Therapy Education:** Provides a listing of courses that may be helpful as the pre-OT student prepares for college.

(2)

What Is Occupational Therapy?

Definition

In 1993, the Representative Assembly of the American Occupational Therapy Association (AOTA) adopted the following definition of OT:

> Occupational therapy is the use of purposeful activity or interventions to achieve functional outcomes. Achieving functional outcomes means to develop or restore the highest possible level of independence of an individual who is limited by a physical injury or illness, a dysfunctional condition, a cognitive impairment, a psychosocial dysfunction, a mental illness, a developmental or learning disability, or an adverse environmental condition.[1]

Brief History of the Profession

OT began as the Society for the Preservation of Occupational Therapy in 1917; the professional association is now known as AOTA. At that time, the profession focused on humane treatment of individuals institutionalized in asylums. Therapists provided purposeful activities for these individuals to promote their well-being. After World War I, OTs were called into action to provide treatment to thousands of injured servicemen, their focus being primarily rehabilitative. A 6-week course was developed to train therapists on the therapeutic use of crafts. World War II saw the profession continuing to provide therapy, addressing the whole person and focusing on psychological as well as physical concerns.

Specialization within the profession began in the 1960s. Currently, the profession has two specialty certification exams administered by the AOTA: pediatrics and neurorehabilitation. In the 1970s, the profession directed its attention to community-based programs in schools and community mental health centers. In the 1980s and 1990s, the profession has continued to promote specialization and expansion of services into a variety of areas and has refocused the profession on occupation.

Where Do Occupational Therapists Work?

- Inpatient, partial hospitalization, and outpatient mental health and substance-abuse treatment centers
- Community mental health centers
- Public or private schools
- Hospital settings, including acute-care, general, or specialized rehabilitation units; pain-management programs; neonatal intensive-care units; outpatient rehabilitation; cardiac rehabilitation; and skilled nursing units
- Nursing homes
- Home-health-care agencies
- Private practice
- Free-standing industrial rehabilitation and work-hardening settings
- Long-term residential facilities for developmentally delayed or mentally challenged persons
- Community reentry facilities
- Physicians' offices
- Orthopedic and hand therapy clinics
- Early intervention programs

What Type of Education Do Occupational Therapists and Certified Occupational Therapy Assistants Receive?

COTAs can enter practice upon completion of an associate degree. OTRs can enter practice after completing a bachelor's degree or entry-level master's degree.

Part of the education of the COTA and OTR includes clinical fieldwork. Individuals may often be able to choose the setting in which they complete their clinical education. Level I clinical education is typically completed during the students' academic coursework. Level II clinical education is typically completed once students have finished all, or a very large portion of, the educational and academic requirements for the degree they are pursuing. Students may complete clinical education in a number of different practice areas. The areas in which OTs practice are presented in this text.

Upon successful completion of either educational program, individuals must successfully pass a national certification exam to practice as a COTA or OTR.

What Tasks Would an Occupational Therapist Perform on a Daily Basis?

Depending on the environment in which they are employed, OTs may:

- Create learning environments for physically challenged children
- Provide purposeful activities to build self-esteem in teens recovering from drug abuse

- Adapt home environments for people dealing with the effects of a stroke
- Analyze job task requirements for an injured worker
- Conduct research to measure effectiveness of treatment activities
- Aid in the growth and development of premature infants
- Fabricate splints and adaptive equipment and devices
- Educate individuals on activity participation that facilitates wellness.[2]

What Are the Philosophical Assumptions in Occupational Therapy?

OT focuses on provision of services to individuals who demonstrate functional limitations in the areas of self-maintenance, productivity, and leisure.[3] OTs assist these individuals in fulfilling their needs through the use of purposeful activity or occupation. The focus of the OT is to develop and maintain function throughout the individual's life. To achieve this, OTs are educated in assessing and treating individual performance deficits. To determine appropriate assessment(s), OTs are guided by theory. Reed identified eight major issues related to theory and OT.[4] These are as follows:

1. Theory assists a profession in defining and describing a specific body of knowledge.
2. A single theory offers specific approaches that can be compared with other theories as well as other professions.
3. Theory guides and directs growth within a profession.
4. Theory assists the OT in articulating a "domain of concern" within the profession. For example, the domain of concern within the profession of OT is the "relationship of occupation to person, environment and health." (p. 521)[4]
5. Theory guides professional decision making within assessment and treatment.
6. Theory within the profession changes with the development of new knowledge as well as with the changes in the health-care system.
7. Theory provides a method for therapists to communicate within as well as outside of the profession of OT.
8. Theory is a method of "translating ideas and hunches into concepts and variables that can be organized systematically and studied." (p. 521)[4]

There are many theories within the profession of OT. Theory guides the practice of OT within the profession.

Employment Options

Currently, OT is one of the fastest-growing professions. By the year 2005, the number of OT positions is expected to increase by 55%.[2]

What Is the Difference Between Occupational Therapy and Physical Therapy?

OT examines the social, psychological, and physical factors that assist a person to become as independent as possible in performing activities necessary to function in home, school, or work environments. Physical therapy (PT) involves treatment focused on helping a person with a physical disability regain movement in affected joints or limbs.[2]

For more information on the comparison between the two professions, read further in this text. Examples are offered comparing the two professions.

Trends in Occupational Therapy

* The fastest-growing areas of practice in OT are home health, private practice, and gerontology.
* The number of universities and community colleges that have OT and OT assistant (OTA) programs is increasing at a rapid pace.
* There is a continued focus on the development of specialization and testing of skills in therapists as evidenced by the AOTA's pediatric and neurorehabilitation specialty examinations as well as the hand therapy certification offered by the American Society of Hand Therapists.
* Advanced assistive technology and life support systems are having an impact on treatment.
* The continued changes in funding for health-care services have been influenced by increased managed care and governmental and legislative changes.
* There is a need for clinical research and outcome studies on the effectiveness of OT.

References

1. American Occupational Therapy Association. (1993). Definition of occupational therapy practice for state regulation. *American Journal of Occupational Therapy*, 47(12), 1117.
2. American Occupational Therapy Association. (1994). Facts about occupational therapy. Bethesda, MD: Author.
3. Reed, K.L., & Sanderson, S.N. (1992). *Concepts of occupational therapy* (3rd ed.). Baltimore, MD: Williams & Wilkins.
4. Reed, K.L. (1997). Theory and frame of reference. In M.E. Neistadt & E.B. Crepeau (Eds.), *Willard and Spackman's occupational therapy* (9th ed.). Philadelphia, PA: Lippincott-Raven.

3

Health Professionals Related to Occupational Therapy

The OT on a rehabilitation team works collaboratively with many other health-care professionals to address client needs. The composition of the treatment team will vary, depending on the type of facility in which an OT is employed. The OT is an integral part of a multidisciplinary treatment team that may include any or all of the following health-care professionals:

- Speech-language pathologists
- Physical therapists (PTs)
- Physical therapist assistants (PTAs)
- Social workers
- Certified therapeutic recreation specialists
- Physician assistants (PAs)
- Dietitians
- Nurses
- Case managers
- Rehabilitation aides and technologists

The following sections will present information regarding the health-care professionals who work collaboratively with the OT to address client issues. The roles and responsibilities of these health-care practitioners, the education required by the respective profession to practice, and the practitioner's professional relationship with the OT on the treatment team will be presented.

Speech-Language Pathologist

Speech-language pathologists provide assessment and treatment to clients with speech, language, voice, or fluency dysfunction.[1] These professionals may also work with individuals who have oral motor problems that may pose difficulties in eating and swallowing. The speech-language pathologist provides direct treatment to clients with communication disorders. According to the American Speech-Language-Hearing Association (ASHA), 1 in 6 Americans has a speech-, language-, or hearing-related disorder.[2] Speech-language pathologists provide treatment to clients who have experienced a stroke or brain injury in order to redevelop the speech and language skills affected by the injury.

When working with children and adolescents, speech-language pathologists provide treatment to address language disorders to improve the students' performance in school. These professionals also offer guidance to individuals who have a language disorder and to their family members to help them deal with the communication impairment of their loved one.[2]

Characteristics that ASHA identifies as important for pursuing a career in this area include an interest in assisting people, a sensitive nature, and tact.

Speech-language pathologists must successfully complete a master's degree in speech-language pathology, 300 to 375 hours of clinical experience under the supervision of an accredited therapist, a national examination, and 9 months of postgraduate experience in a clinical setting.[1] In a few states, individuals with a bachelor of science degree may work in a school setting with children with communication disorders. They must be certified by the state educational agency, however, and are often given the title of special education teacher.

The professional outlook for these professionals is positive. ASHA indicates that greater public awareness and understanding of communication disorders, early diagnosis of speech-language and hearing disorders, and an aging population concerned with hearing disorders resulting from occupational responsibilities all provide a bright future for individuals who desire to pursue a professional career as a speech-language pathologist.[2]

Speech-language pathologists typically work as part of a multidisciplinary team with OTs. These professionals work collaboratively to assess clients' oral motor skills and level of cognition. Speech-language pathologists provide treatment in conjunction with an OT, depending on the diagnosis of the client with whom they are working. Within treatment sessions the speech-language pathologist may address the clients' comprehension of instructions as well as their responses to verbal directions while the OT engages them in functional, purposeful activities that have meaning for the clients and address their functional limitations.

For more information on speech-language pathology as a profession, contact:

American Speech-Language-Hearing Association
10801 Rockville Pike
Rockville, MD 29852
Phone: 800-498-2071; 301-897-5700
TTY: 301-897-0157
FAX: 301-571-0457
Web site: http://www.asha.org

Physical Therapist and Physical Therapy Assistant

According to the *Dictionary of Occupational Titles*, published by the Bureau of Labor Statistics, a PT's role and function include:

- Improving mobility
- Relieving pain
- Preventing or limiting permanent physical disabilities in individuals who have experienced an injury or disease process[3]

PTs and PTAs frequently provide treatment for the following diagnoses:

- Cerebral palsy
- Nerve injuries
- Amputations
- Head injuries
- Multiple sclerosis
- Fractures
- Low back injuries and pain
- Arthritis
- Heart disease
- Function and independence affected by some type of accident

Many PTs choose to specialize in a specific practice area. Specific specialty practice areas within the profession of PT include:

- Pediatrics
- Geriatrics
- Orthopedics
- Sports medicine
- Neurology
- Cardiopulmonary therapy[3]

Treatment provided by a PT begins after the therapist completes an evaluation to determine the patient's level of function. The therapist may test an individual's range of motion, strength, and ability to engage in functional activity. Upon completion of the assessment, the PT will develop a plan of treatment. The PTA may carry out this plan of treatment, including specific procedures identified by the PT.[3] Methods that PTs may employ in the treatment of dysfunction may include range-of-motion activities and exercises to improve balance, coordination, and endurance. PTs also use physical agent modalities. These modalities include heat, cold, electrical stimulation, and ultrasound. PTs are also responsible for educating individuals in correct body positioning and the use of crutches, wheelchairs, and prostheses.

The American Physical Therapy Association (APTA) encourages students interested in pursuing a career in PT to obtain education at the postbaccalaureate level.[4] The APTA believes that this level of education prepares PTs to address the changing medical needs of individuals as the arena of health care continues to grow and expand. PT education includes basic science courses and specialized science courses in biomechanics, neuroanatomy, human growth and development, pathology of disease and trauma, evaluation and assessment techniques, treatment methods, and research.

In addition to academic education, students are required to complete clinical experience. According to the APTA, 60 weeks of classroom and laboratory experience, as well as 24 weeks of clinical experience, are covered in 2 or 3 academic or calendar years in a professional PT curriculum.[5] The PTA works under the direct supervision of a PT and assists the PT in carrying out a successful plan of treatment.

An individual wishing to pursue a career in PT should possess the following characteristics:

- Strong interpersonal skills
- Compassion
- A desire to understand and explain disabilities to clients and their families
- Manual dexterity and physical stamina (to successfully complete the duties of a PT)

The PT and OT often work collaboratively on a multidisciplinary team, providing assessment and treatment for functional limitations in a variety of client diagnoses. For example, in evaluating a client in a pediatric setting, the PT may address gross motor evaluation whereas the OT may complete the fine motor evaluation. However, an OT is trained and qualified to complete the gross motor assessment as well.

The type of facility or setting and the individual therapist's training and specialty areas may determine many differences between the professionals' responsibilities. Typically, in most settings, PTs may have a limited involvement in assisting the client in completion of activities of daily living. PTs may not use purposeful activity, which is a hallmark of OT. PTs typically do not use crafts for treatment of client deficits. Additionally, PTs are not frequently involved with individuals diagnosed with mental illness unless the client presents a secondary physical limitation.

For more information on the profession of PT contact:

American Physical Therapy Association
111 N. Fairfax St.
Alexandria, VA 22314-1488
Phone: 703-684-APTA
FAX: 703-684-7343
Web site: http://www.apta.org

Social Worker

According to the National Association of Social Workers, the primary mission of the profession of social work is to promote human well-being as well as to assist in meeting the basic needs of all individuals, with particular attention focused on individuals who are vulnerable, oppressed, and living in poverty.[6]

A social worker is another professional with whom an OT may interact to provide effective care to clients. Social workers provide direct counseling to clients and their families, as well as address problems the clients may face, including:

- Lack of housing
- Employment
- Inability to manage finances
- Substance abuse
- Unplanned pregnancy
- Antisocial behavior[3]

Social workers may provide individual or family counseling to address problem areas as well as provide information and resources about community services to fulfill the client's identified needs. In addition to counseling, these professionals may arrange for a client to receive specific services and may follow the client through provision of these services to determine their effectiveness.

Many social workers specialize in a certain area of practice. Some areas that social workers may specialize in include:

- Child welfare and family services
- School social work
- Psychotherapy in community mental-health settings
- Public relief agencies
- Child or adult protective services investigating suspected abuse
- Crisis intervention within a homeless shelter or battered women's shelter
- Hospital-based programs
- Employee assistance programs[3]

A bachelor's degree is required for social work practice in most areas for most positions. A master's degree in social work, however, is most often necessary in health and mental health settings.[3] A bachelor of science degree typically prepares an individual to perform the direct service duties of a case worker or group worker. This degree includes coursework in social work practice, social welfare, human behavior, community environment, and research methods. The bachelor of social work degree also requires the individual to complete 400 hours of supervised field experience.[3]

A master of social work (MSW) degree includes coursework in assessment, case management, and supervision. Typically, an MSW program occurs over a course of 2 years and includes 900 hours of supervised field experience. Entry into an MSW program does not require completion of a bachelor of social work degree. It is important to note, however, that coursework completed in psychology, biology, sociology, economics, political science, history, social anthropology, urban studies, and social work is strongly suggested.[3]

An individual who wishes to pursue a career in social work should possess the following characteristics:

- Emotional maturity
- Objectivity
- Sensitivity to people and varied problems

- Ability to work independently
- Ability to maintain a good working relationship with a variety of individuals from various ethnic and cultural backgrounds.[3]

A social worker and OT may collaborate to provide effective care to clients in a number of areas. For example, an OT may complete a home evaluation with a client prior to discharge from the hospital. During the evaluation, the OT may determine that the client is unsafe while cooking. In all other areas of the home evaluation, the client demonstrates independence. Upon return to the hospital, the OT alerts the social worker to her or his concerns. The social worker assists the client in determining what services would be appropriate to meet the client's safety needs. The alternatives the social worker may present to the client could include Meals on Wheels, congregate group meal site attendance, or a homemaker to come to the client's home to assist in meal preparation. In this situation, the OT identified a deficit in the client's living environment. With the assistance of the social worker, the OT was able to assist the client in obtaining the least restrictive discharge environment.

For more information on the profession of social work contact:

National Association of Social Workers
IC-Career Information
750 First Street NE
Suite 700
Washington, DC 20002-4241
Phone: 202-408-8600
FAX: 202-336-8311
TTY: 202-408-8396
Web site: http://www.socialworkers.org

Recreational Therapist

Recreational therapists use activities to provide treatment for or to maintain the physical, mental, and emotional well-being of the clients.[3] Activities that a recreational therapist may use as part of treatment may include, but are not limited to:

- Community outings
- Sports
- Games
- Arts and crafts
- Drama
- Dance
- Music

These activities are used to address the client's ability to socialize, develop self-confidence, and, most frequently, address and remediate areas of functional limitation because of a disease or disability. It is of utmost importance that recreational therapists not be confused with recreation workers. The primary difference between the two oc-

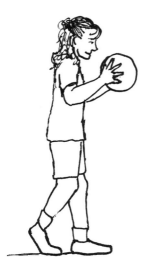
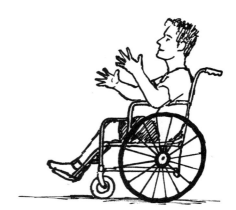

cupations is that recreation workers organize activities primarily for enjoyment, whereas recreational therapists use activities for treatment of deficits or dysfunction.[3]

Recreational therapists may be employed in hospital and rehabilitation settings, as well as in nursing homes, community-based mental-health treatment centers, special-education programs, and a variety of residential treatment settings.

Duties performed by a recreational therapist include assessment, development, and implementation of therapeutic activity programs addressing functional limitations identified during the assessment. For example, a client who demonstrates problems with socialization because of a stroke and accompanying language problems may be assisted in learning how to play a board game independently. Of primary importance to the recreational therapist is that the program that he or she develops must address the functional limitations the client is experiencing as well as meet the client's needs and interests.[3]

The education required for a recreational therapist is a bachelor of science degree in therapeutic recreation. Courses for this degree include:

- Clinical skills
- Interpersonal helping skills
- Program development and management
- Professional ethics and issues
- Anatomy and physiology
- Abnormal psychology
- Medical terminology
- Study of disease and disability
- Assessment
- Referral
- Use of adaptive equipment and technology

In addition to academic coursework, recreational therapy students are required to complete 360 hours of clinical internship under the supervision of a certified therapeutic recreation specialist.[3] An associate degree in recreational therapy or qualifying experience may be acceptable in a nursing home setting to perform the duties of an activity director.

Characteristics necessary for success in this profession include understanding and comfort in working with people who have a variety of disabilities and functional limitations:

- Patience
- Tact and persuasion
- Imagination and determination since recreational therapists frequently adapt activities to meet clients' needs
- Physical coordination for demonstrating and participating in recreational events

A recreational therapist and OT may interact to facilitate independence in client function in a number of areas. The two professionals may work collaboratively in community outings with individual clients or groups of clients. The recreational therapist may work with the client to plan the outing and address possible accessibility issues because the client is in a wheelchair. The OT may work with clients to address cognitive areas of money management as well as sequencing steps of a portion of an activity, for example, transferring from a wheelchair to a theater seat.

For more information about the profession of recreational therapy contact:

American Therapeutic Recreation Association
C.O. Associated Management Systems
P.O. Box 15215
Hattiesburg, MS 39402-5215
Phone: 601-264-3413
FAX: 601-264-3337
Web site: http://www.atra-tr.org

National Therapeutic Recreation Society
22377 Belmont Ridge Rd.
Ashburn, VA 20148
Phone: 703-858-0784
FAX: 703-858-0794
Web site: http://www.nrpa.org

Physician Assistant

The primary responsibility of a PA is to support and assist a physician in completion of patient care responsibilities.[3] It is important, however, not to confuse the profession of PA with medical assistant. These two professions have different responsibilities. PAs are trained to complete routine physicals, make diagnoses, and provide therapeutic and preventative treatment under the direct supervision of a physician. These

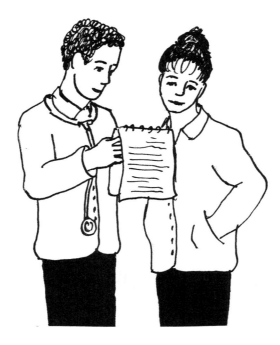

professionals are also trained to complete medical histories, perform patient examinations, order and interpret laboratory and diagnostic tests, and develop a preliminary diagnosis. In many states, PAs may also prescribe medication.

In many rural areas, PAs may be the only medical professionals available to the residents of that area. PAs may work in general medicine, pediatrics, and family practice. Some professionals, however, may specialize in areas such as general surgery, emergency medicine, orthopedics, and geriatrics.[7]

Education for entry into the profession includes completion of a 4-year degree program. Typically, students complete 2 years of coursework in English, biology, chemistry, math, social sciences, and psychology. Many individuals who pursue careers in this area have past work experience as emergency medical technicians or other health-care professionals, such as nurses. The PA's education includes coursework in the following areas:

- Biochemistry
- Nutrition
- Anatomy and physiology
- Microbiology
- Clinical pharmacology
- Clinical medicine
- Ethics
- Geriatrics
- Home health care
- Disease prevention

Students are additionally required to complete clinical rotations in several areas. These areas include:

- Family medicine
- Ambulatory medicine
- Surgery
- Obstetrics and gynecology
- Geriatrics
- Emergency medicine
- Internal medicine
- Psychiatry
- Pediatrics[3]

Individuals wishing to pursue a career as a PA should possess the following characteristics:

- Leadership
- Self-assurance
- Emotional maturity
- A desire to pursue life-long learning, because continuing education is a requirement for this profession[3]

A PA may interact with OTs by referring clients to therapy for assessment and treatment. The OT may provide the PA with evaluative information that may assist the PA in making a diagnosis and planning for effective treatment for the client.

For more information on a profession as a PA contact:

American Academy of Physician Assistants
950 N. Washington St.
Alexandria, VA 22314
Phone: 703-836-2272
FAX: 703-531-1558
Web site: http://www.aapa.org

Dietitian

The professional role and function of a dietitian are to plan nutrition programs and supervise the preparation and serving of meals.[3] These professionals evaluate, prevent, and treat illness through the promotion of healthy eating habits. They prescribe, under the supervision and guidance of a physician, diets that may include modifications of reduced salt, sugar, fat, and protein. There are multiple areas in which dietitians may practice. They may supervise food service activities for various institutions such as hospitals and school systems. Dietitians may also be involved in the promotion of positive lifestyle through examination and education of eating habits as well as research. The primary areas of clinical practice for dietitians are:

- Clinical
- Community

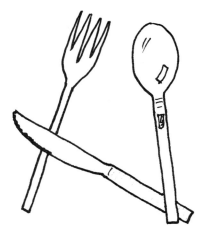

- Management
- Consultation[3]

Individuals wishing to pursue a career in dietetics are required to complete a bachelor's degree in dietetics, foods and nutrition, food service systems management, or a related area. Coursework typically includes courses in

- Food
- Nutrition
- Management
- Chemistry
- Biology
- Microbiology
- Math
- Statistics
- Computer science
- Physiology
- Psychology
- Sociology
- Economics

Supervised practice is an additional requirement for this profession. The practice may be obtained during the academic preparation within a 4-year program or 900 hours of supervised practice at an American Dietetics Association (ADA)–accredited internship site.[3] To become a dietetic technician, an individual must complete an associate degree in this area. Dietetic technicians collaborate with and work under the direct supervision of a dietitian.[8]

Characteristics of an individual desiring to pursue a career in dietetics include:

- A sincere interest in food and nutrition
- A desire to work with people
- Motivation

- Initiative
- Good judgment
- Thorough understanding of human nature
- Problem-solving abilities[8]

A dietitian and OT may work collaboratively to address feeding and eating issues. The team of professionals may address types and consistency of foods that would best enable a client to feed herself or himself. These professionals may work together to educate the client on appropriate food selection according to their diagnosis. The dietitian may educate the client on appropriate food choice. The OT will reinforce the education provided by the dietitian and assist the client in preparation of the food in an independent manner by adapting the method in which the food was prepared, depending on the client's functional limitations, or issuing adaptive equipment.

For more information on a career as a dietitian contact:

The American Dietetic Association
216 W. Jackson Blvd.
Chicago, IL 60606-6995
Phone: 312-899-0040
FAX: 312-899-1979
Web site: http://www.eatright.org

Nurse

Registered nurses provide care for individuals who are sick or injured, promote wellness, and assist individuals to stay healthy.[3] Nurses provide holistic care, addressing not only the physical but also the social, emotional, and mental needs of their clients. Nurses observe clients, assess their condition, record symptoms, assess progress with treatment, administer medications, and assist physicians. Additionally, nurses work to educate family members regarding the client's condition and

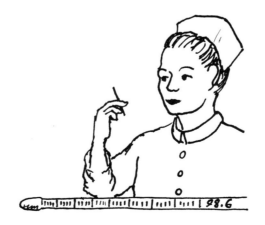

course of treatment. Within the profession of nursing, individual states regulate the specific procedures that nurses may perform. Nurses may be employed in hospitals, physician's offices, home health care settings, nursing homes, public health agencies, and industrial settings.

Individuals who desire to specialize may pursue additional education and become nurse practitioners. Other areas of specialized practice in nursing include clinical nurse specialist, nurse anesthetist, and certified nurse midwife.[3]

Education for nurses may occur at several levels. An individual may pursue an associate degree, a diploma nursing program, or a bachelor of science in nursing. Associate nursing degree programs offered at community or junior colleges typically require 2 years for completion. Diploma programs offered at hospitals and medical centers are often structured for completion in 2 to 3 years. Universities offering a bachelor of science in nursing frequently structure the academic coursework over 4 to 5 years. Coursework includes:

- Anatomy and physiology
- Microbiology
- Chemistry
- Nutrition
- Psychology
- Microbiology
- Nursing

In addition to academic coursework, students are required to complete supervised clinical experience. This clinical experience may include such areas as:

- Pediatrics
- Psychiatry
- Maternity
- General medicine
- Surgery[3]

Qualities an individual must possess to be successful in the profession of nursing include:

- Caring
- Sympathetic sensitivity
- The ability to accept responsibility
- The ability to follow orders precisely
- The ability to determine when further assistance is needed

For more information on a nursing career contact:

American Nurses Association
600 Maryland Avenue, SW
Washington, DC 20024-2571
Phone: 800-669-1656; 212-989-9393
FAX: 212-989-3710
Web site: http://www.nln.org

Case Manager

Case management is not a profession per se. Rather, it is a practice area within a variety of professions.[9] Case management dates back to the 1900s, when nurses and social workers coordinated services to ensure continuity of care for the clients they served. Currently, case management services are provided by a variety of professionals in a vast number of different practice settings.[9]

In 1993, the credential of certified case manager was introduced and sponsored by the Certification of Insurance Rehabilitation Specialists Commission. The philosophy of case management is to assist individuals in obtaining an optimal level of health and wellness. Through the provision of case management services, many other systems outside the individual benefit. The individual's support system, health-care delivery system, and reimbursement sources all benefit. The case manager assists the client in obtaining an optimal level of health and wellness by:

- Promoting client autonomy
- Serving as a client advocate
- Communicating with various agencies and support services
- Educating
- Identifying service resources and service facilitation

The case manager communicates with the entire treatment team to coordinate and facilitate continuity of care and services for the client. The role of the case manager is also to ensure that services provided are not duplicated or fragmented in any manner.[9]

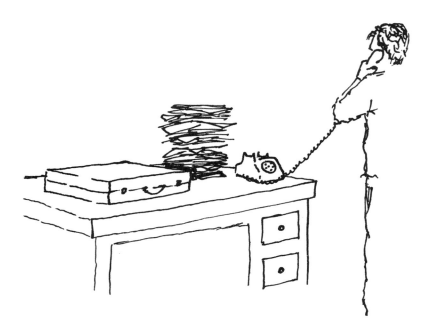

Within case management there is a process of functions or duties the case manager performs. These duties include identification of clients, information gathering, planning, reporting, obtaining approval for services, coordination of services and plan of action, follow-up, and evaluation.

The characteristics of an individual who may choose to pursue a career in case management include:

- An ability to focus on individual as well as societal needs
- An ability to empower individuals to make independent decisions
- Responsibility
- Accountability[9]

An OT may perform the duties of a case manager, depending on the setting in which the therapist practices. Additionally, an OT may collaborate with a case manager to ensure that the appropriate type and level of services are provided to the client.

For more information on certified case management contact:

Commission for Case Management Certification
1835 Rohlwing Road
Suite D
Rolling Meadows, IL, 60008
Phone: 847-818-0292

Certified Nurse Assistant and Rehabilitation Aide

These paraprofessionals are trained at vocational training centers or community colleges to assist nurses and other health-care professionals. Typically, they are involved in daily direct patient care and may carry out various treatment plans under the direct supervision of a nurse or other health-care professionals.

Education for these paraprofessionals typically includes coursework in:

- Basic nursing skills
- Restorative services
- Personal care skills
- Safety
- Emergency-care issues

Students are educated in the importance of addressing clients' needs while consistently attending to their mental and emotional needs, overall safety, and well-being. Depending on the program and facility providing the education, the coursework may be covered in a typical classroom as well as in laboratory settings. Supervised clinical experience may be required as well.

Individuals trained in nursing assistance or rehabilitation may have to complete an examination to become certified, depending on the state in which they plan to practice.

Characteristics required of individuals who wish to pursue this career include:

- Compassion
- Sympathy
- An ability to manage multiple tasks simultaneously
- Patience
- Physical stamina for transferring clients
- A desire to work as an integral part of a multidisciplinary treatment team

Certified nurse assistants and rehabilitation aides may assist OTs in preparing clients for scheduled treatment sessions, transporting clients to and from treatment sessions, and performing some types of treatment under the direct supervision of the OT.

For more information on certified nurse assistant programs or rehabilitation aide training, contact your local community college, local junior college, or vocational training center.

References

1. Bureau of Labor Statistics. (1996). Occupational outlook handbook. *Bureau of Labor Statistics Homepage* [On-line]. Available: http://stats.bls.gov
2. American Speech-Language-Hearing Association. (1996). Career information. *American Speech-Language-Hearing Association Homepage* [On-line]. Available: http://www.asha.org/career.htm
3. Bureau of Labor Statistics. (1997). *Dictionary of Occupational Titles* [On-line]. Available: http://stats.bls.gov/oco/ocodict/htm
4. American Physical Therapy Association. (1997). General information for students. *American Physical Therapy Association Homepage* [On-line]. Available: http://www.apta.org/education/gen_info.html#physical_therapy_education
5. American Physical Therapy Association. (1994). The commonalties and differences between the professions of physical therapy and occupational therapy. *American Physical Therapy Association House of Delegates Manual.* Alexandria, VA: Author.
6. National Association of Social Workers. (1993). *Code of ethics.* Washington, DC: Author.
7. American Academy of Physician Assistants. (1997). Facts at a glance. *American Academy of Physician Assistants Homepage* [On-line]. Available: http://www.aapa.org/geninfo1.htm
8. American Dietetics Association. (1997). ADA: Education/experience requirements. *American Dietetic Association Homepage* [On-line]. Available: http://www.eatright.org
9. Cassell, J.L., Mulkey, S.W., & Engen, C. (1997). Systematic practice: Case and caseload management. In D.R. Maki & T.F. Riggar (Eds.), *Rehabilitation counseling: Profession and practice.* New York: Springer.

$$\widehat{4}$$

What Is the Difference Between Occupational Therapy and Physical Therapy?

Definition of Occupational Therapy

Occupational Therapy is the use of purposeful activity or interventions to achieve functional outcomes. Achieving functional outcomes means to develop or restore the highest possible level of independence of an individual who is limited by a physical injury or illness, a dysfunctional condition, a cognitive impairment, a psychosocial dysfunction, a mental illness, a developmental or learning disability, or an adverse environmental condition. Assessment means the use of skilled observation or evaluation by the administration and interpretation of standardized or nonstandardized tests and measurements to identify areas for occupational therapy services. Occupational therapy services include but are not limited to: assessment, treatment and education of or consultation with the individual, family or other persons; or interventions directed toward developing, improving or restoring daily living skills, work readiness, or work performance, play skills or leisure capacities, or enhancing educational performance skills or neuromuscular functioning or range of motion; or emotional, motivational, cognitive, or psychosocial components of performance. These services may require assessment of the need for and the use of interventions such as the design, development, adaptation, application, or training in the use of assistive technology such as selected orthotic or prosthetic devices; the application of physical agent modalities as an adjunct to or in preparation for purposeful activity; the use of ergonomic principles; the adaptation of environments and processes to enhance functional performance; or the promotion of health and wellness.[1]

Definition of Physical Therapy

Physical therapy is the assessment, evaluation, and treatment and prevention of physical disability, movement dysfunction and pain resulting from injury, disease, disability, or other health related conditions. Physical therapy includes: the performance and interpretation of tests and measurements to assess pathophysiological, pathomechanical, electrophysiological, ergonomic, and developmental deficits of body systems to determine diagnosis, treatment, prognosis and prevention; the planning, administration and modification of therapeutic coordination, joint mobility, flexibility, pain, healing and repair, and functional activities in daily living skills, including work; and the provision of consultative, educational, research and other advisory services. The therapeutic interventions may include, but are not limited to, the use of therapeutic exercises with or without assistive devices, physical agents, electricity, manual procedures such as joint and soft tissue mobilization, neuromuscular reeducation, bronchopulmonary hygiene and ambulation/gait training. (p. 123)[2]

Education and Professional Training

An individual may enter OT at two levels: baccalaureate degree or professional master's degree.[3] The current trend in the profession is toward the development of a professional master's degree. A typical program awarding a baccalaureate degree spans 4 years plus a minimum of 6 months of supervised full time clinical fieldwork education. An OT assistant (OTA) candidate would work toward an associate degree, which typically includes supervised clinical education of 2 months, on completion of the last academic term.[3]

PT education includes 72 credits of preprofessional educational content and 90 hours of academic and clinical education. According to the APTA, the average time in direct classroom experience is 60 weeks, with 24 weeks of clinical education occurring over the course of 2 to 3 academic years. The majority of PT programs award a professional master's degree.[2] PTAs are awarded an associate of applied science degree upon successful completion of 50 weeks of academic experience and 20 weeks of clinical education.

Licensure and Examination Procedures

In the United States, upon successful completion of each level of education, OT, PT, OTA, and PTA, the individual is eligible to sit for a national certification examination. The purpose of these examinations is to assess the individual's competence prior to initial certification. To sit for the examination, an individual must have been graduated from an accredited program of OT or PT. Each profession has its own supervising agency to monitor this process. Within the profession of OT, the National Board for Certification in Occupational Therapy (NBCOT) monitors the examination process. Within the profession of PT, the Federation of State Boards of Physical Therapy monitors the examination process.[2]

In the United States, each state regulates therapy services differently. It is the responsibility of professional practitioners to obtain and comply with all professional practice regulations for the state in which they wish to practice. Each state may have different requirements for continuing education to demonstrate continued competency and relicensure.

Specialization in Practice

The AOTA currently supervises two specialty certifications for the practicing OT. These specialty certifications are for pediatrics and neurorehabilitation. To obtain specialty certification in either one of these practice areas, the practicing therapist must meet criteria established by the AOTA and the Specialty Certification Board as well as successfully complete a certification examination. It is important to note that these specialty certification examinations are completed on a voluntary basis. OTs are encouraged to participate in this advanced credentialing process, but it is not mandatory for practice.

The profession of PT has established specialist certification programs that assess and acknowledge advanced clinical skills and experience in the following areas: cardiopulmonary, clinical, electrophysiological, geriatric, neurological, orthopedic, pediatric, and sports PT.[2]

Roles in Practice

The PT is responsible for the following roles, regardless of the type of setting in which services are provided:

- Screening of patients for appropriateness of service
- Initial assessment, interpretation, and diagnosis for PT services
- Identification of roles and responsibilities of tasks that can be completed by the PTA and those that must be completed by the PT
- Delegation of tasks deemed appropriate to the PTA as well as to other support staff, including PT technicians or rehabilitation aides
- Consistent review and reevaluation of the treatment process and adjustment of the treatment plan according to client level of function or dysfunction
- Plan for client discharge and establishment of a home program or other appropriate follow-up referrals[2]

Within the professions of OT and PT, the following roles may be fulfilled by the practitioner:

- Practitioner
- Educator
- Fieldwork educator
- Supervisor
- Administrator
- Consultant
- Fieldwork coordinator
- Faculty
- Program director
- Researcher or scholar
- Entrepreneur[4]

An OT is responsible for the following roles as an entry-level practitioner:

- Initiation of referrals when appropriate
- Completion of client screening to determine appropriateness of service provision
- Evaluation of client function and interpretation of evaluation data to complete effective treatment planning
- Development and collaboration with other health-care professionals to meet client goals for improvement in function and development of independence
- Adaptation of the task and of the environment or prescription of adaptive equipment, depending on the client's level of function, to facilitate client independence in activities of daily living
- Critical examination of client progress toward identified goals and modification of established treatment plan in response to client progress or potential lack of progress
- Communication and provision of ongoing education and understanding regarding the client's progress and condition to other health-care team members; the client; and the client's family, significant other, and caregiver(s)
- Determination that the client has obtained the maximal benefit of treatment and termination of therapeutic services
- Completion of discharge documentation, formulation and instruction of client and significant others on recommendations, and follow-up referrals for other appropriate services
- Completion of documentation as required by agency, reimbursers, and practice setting[2]

That's All Fine and Good, But How About an Example?

The roles and responsibilities of PTs and OTs are clearly defined. Depending on the setting, however, they may work collaboratively on similar issues or areas of dysfunction or they may address very different areas of function.

In a geriatric setting, a PT may evaluate clients' lower extremity function—in other words, bed mobility, gait, and transfer ability. For the same patients and setting, the OT may evaluate upper extremity function, including range of motion and ability to complete functional activities of daily living, such as the clients' ability to wash their faces and hair and brush their teeth. An OT may also evaluate cognitive and perceptual skills. OTs and PTs may work collaboratively to address the client's balance and trunk control. Some PTs, however, may also address dysfunction of the upper extremity within the treatment session. The most important point to remember is that these two professions must work collaboratively to address and remediate the client's functional deficits. In some settings, OTs address bed mobility; in other settings, bed mobility is the responsibility of the PT. Of utmost importance is that the professional provide necessary services to the client while performing within the scope of practice.

Typically, PTs do not use purposeful activities, such as crafts, and do not work with clients diagnosed with mental illness unless the client presents with a secondary physical limitation that would warrant a PT referral. OTs, on the other hand, use functional purposeful activities and crafts that are considered to be the foundation of the profession. The profession of OT began with therapists working with individuals hospitalized in psychiatric facilities.[5]

References

1. American Occupational Therapy Association. (1993). Definition of occupational therapy practice for state regulation. *American Journal of Occupational Therapy*, 47(12), 1117.
2. American Physical Therapy Association. (1994). The commonalities and differences between the professions of physical therapy and occupational therapy. *American Physical Therapy Association House of Delegates Manual*. Alexandria, VA: Author.
3. American Occupational Therapy Association. (1991). Essentials and guidelines for an accredited educational program for the occupational therapist. *American Journal of Occupational Therapy, 45*(12), 1077–1084.
4. American Occupational Therapy Association. (1996). *Reference manual of the official documents of the American Occupational Therapy Association* (6th ed.). Bethesda, MD: Author.
5. Reed, K.L., & Sanderson, S.N. (1992). *Concepts of occupational therapy* (3rd ed.). Baltimore, MD: Williams & Wilkins.

$$\boxed{5}$$

How Do I Decide if Occupational Therapy Is the Right Career for Me?

There are a number of things you need to consider when exploring whether OT is the right career for you. The American Occupational Therapy Association (AOTA) identifies career development as an ongoing process that involves planning and examining individual circumstances, interests, and ethical considerations.[1] The steps in this career investigation include assessing skills and interests, setting goals, completing a thorough examination of the profession via exploration of the social and political environment, examining educational demands for each area of the profession, and making a decision.[1]

Career Placement and Career Exploration Offices

The assessment process can be completed in a number of different ways. Many colleges and universities have career placement or career exploration offices. The staff working in these offices is trained to administer tests that determine individual needs and preferences with regard to careers.

Gain a Thorough Understanding of the Profession

Another important part of assessment is having a thorough understanding of OT as a profession. Many individuals "think" they know what OT is, although they may never have observed an OT or received OT services. A thorough understanding comes only with experience.

Information Gathering

Once you understand the nature of OT, you can gather more information about the profession via numerous avenues. There is a wide variety of valuable information about OT on the Worldwide Web. Search using the terms "occupational therapy" or "occupational therapist." Another option for gaining more information about the profession is by contacting a national association:

American Occupational Therapy Association
4720 Montgomery Lane
P.O. Box 31220
Bethesda, MD 20824-1220
Phone: 800-SAY-AOTA
Web site: http://www.aota.org

Canadian Association of Occupational Therapy
Carleton Technology & Training Centre
Suite 3400
1125 Colonel By Drive
Ottawa, ON, K1S5R1
Phone: 800-434-CAOT
Web site: http://www.caot.ca

Refer to Appendix A for additional information. National associations provide a variety of printed information about choosing OT as a career or considering OT as a second career.

If you are still interested after you have completed your reading and research, it would be beneficial to meet with an OT to discuss his or her roles and responsibilities. This manual is designed to assist you with the observation experience process. On the following pages, there are sample questions to ask the OT with whom you meet prior to beginning your observation experience.

Self-Assessment

In addition to furthering your understanding about the profession, the AOTA suggests that you complete a thorough self-assessment.[1] Within this self-assessment, it is beneficial to address the following:

- How you receive feedback
- How you relate to a variety of individuals from different cultures
- What you feel are your strengths and weaknesses

It is important to be objective during the self-assessment process. You may seek information from teachers, current and past employers, peers, and family members. From a broader perspective, examine current family obligations, living preferences, and financial resources because these areas may be affected should you choose to pursue an education in OT.[1]

Within this book, a professional behavior checklist and professional feedback forms are provided to assist in completion of the self-assessment. If you choose to pursue a career in OT, keep in mind that self-assessment assisted in guiding you to this decision. Self-assessment is not a one-step process; it is important to continue the process throughout your professional career.

Establishing Realistic Goals

Once you have completed the assessment process, it is essential to establish realistic goals related to your pursuit of this career. You might establish goals such as the following:

- Contact AOTA for a current listing of professional and technical educational programs
- Read further in this manual to prepare yourself for a variety of observation and learning experiences
- Contact educational institutions for information about admissions
- Review the questions that follow and interview an OT or COTA for more information about the profession
- Determine what additional observation experiences are available to you and contact the facilities and supervising OT or COTA

Questions for an Occupational Therapist—Career Exploration and Assessment Phase

What do you like about your profession?

Could you offer me some advice or direction about how I might best prepare for entering an educational program in OT?

Could you give me examples of what you like about your job?

What are some things you dislike about your job?

How did you find out about the profession of OT?

What do you think is the outlook for the job market for OTs and COTAs?

What are some tasks that you perform on a daily basis as part of your job?

Reference

1. American Occupational Therapy Association. (1996). *Reference manual of the official documents of the American Occupational Therapy Association* (6th ed.). Bethesda, MD: Author.

6

Current Working Conditions Within the Profession of Occupational Therapy

It is important for the pre-OT student to understand that statistics regarding the profession change quite rapidly. Additionally, it is important to note that the information contained here may vary depending on the type of setting in which the therapist is employed, as well as the geographic location of employment.

What Is the Job Outlook for the Profession?

Currently, the job outlook for OTs is excellent, and it is anticipated that the profession will continue to grow. It is believed that the largest areas of growth will be within rehabilitation and long-term care. As the "Baby Boomers" age and medical technology continues to expand, life-span services will be required to serve these individuals. Another area of increased growth and need is within home health care. Because individuals are being discharged from hospitals at a faster rate than ever before, additional services may be required within the home environment.[1]

What Is the Salary for Occupational Therapists?

According to information from a 1994 survey, therapists earn a median annual salary of $39,634, based on a 40-hour work week. The minimum salary rate is $33,728; the average maximum salary is $49,392. Therapists who work different shifts or in specific practice areas may be compensated for advanced skills or training. The survey also identified that therapists who worked in private practice reported earnings greater than those just mentioned.[1]

Salaries will vary depending on the type of practice setting and the geographic location. Additionally, when considering salary, it is important to examine not only the wage but also the fringe benefits. These benefits may include medical and dental insurance, malpractice insurance, continuing education, and travel benefits, as well as many other items that may be offered by the employer.

What Other Professions Are Related?

Depending on the setting, an OT may work with some of the following related professionals: dietitians, speech-language pathologists and audiologists, PTs, recreational therapists, teachers, music therapists, creative arts therapists, art therapists, vocational rehabilitation counselors, certified addiction counselors, medical doctors, nurses, certified nurse assistants, rehabilitation aides, psychologists, physicians, psychiatrists, and social workers.[1]

Where Are Occupational Therapy Services Provided?

OT services are provided at inpatient and outpatient rehabilitation centers, nursing care centers, schools, hospitals, mental health units, community mental health centers, hospices, and industrial rehabilitation settings and as part of home-health and substance-abuse treatment programs.

How Can I Find Out More About Occupational Therapy?

In the United States contact the American Occupational Therapy Association at 301-652-2682, http://www.aota.org

In Canada contact the Canadian Association of Occupational Therapists at 800-434-CAOT, http://www.caot.ca

Reference

1. Bureau of Labor Statistics. (1997). *Dictionary of Occupational Titles* [On-line]. Available: http://stats.bls.gov./oco/ocodict/htm

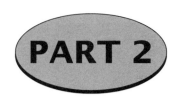

Education

OTR and COTA Role Delineation

For more information on OTR and COTA role delineation, see the *Reference Manual of the Official Documents of the American Occupational Therapy Association* (6th ed.) (1996).

OTR	COTA
Referral	
Generally makes the decision on what clients the COTA will treat	Generally receives referrals from an OTR, but an experienced COTA may help screen for appropriate referrals
May initiate appropriate referrals or screen patients for referrals	
Evaluations	
	Assists the OTR with data collection for evaluation under OTR supervision
Completes evaluations and determines treatment plan	Develops goals for treatment under OTR supervision
	An experienced COTA may complete standardized evaluations under OTR supervision
Treatment	
Develops treatment plans with goals	Provides treatment for patients under OTR supervision
Completes a variety of treatments for any area or age	Documents treatment
Adapts the environment, treatment technique, and equipment as needed for the individual	Adapts treatment for patient with OTR collaboration
Collaborates with interdisciplinary team and family or caregivers	

OTR	COTA
Supervision	
Provides supervision for other therapists, therapist assistants, staff, and students	Requires supervision by an OTR (refer to individual state regulations for exactly how much supervision is required)
Requires routine to minimal supervision, depending on her or his experience level	May help supervise other COTAs, OTA students, volunteers, and staff with direction by an OTR

$$\boxed{8}$$

How to Compare Occupational Therapy Schools

Selecting a school for your OT career can be very difficult in view of the many factors to be considered. There are often at least three applicants for every spot. Because of the competitiveness, many choose to apply to more than one school at a time. Here are some ideas to consider.

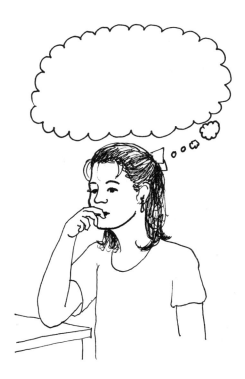

Location

Would you prefer a school close to where you are living, or can you relocate? What is the cost of tuition for applicants who live within the state versus out-of-state applicants? What are the features of the neighborhood surrounding the school? Is housing available on campus? Is it available for new or transfer students? What kind of transportation options do you have or need for getting to school and the various clinical experience sites?

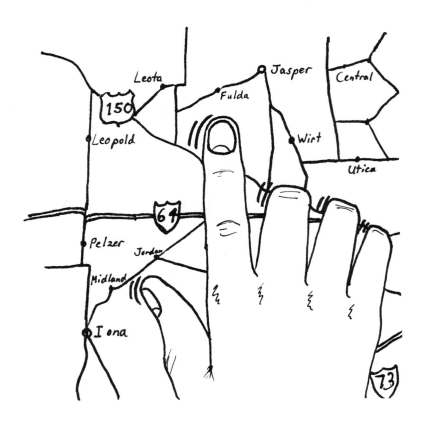

Cost

What is the total estimated tuition for the schooling? What financial aid programs are available? Would you have time to work while you go to school? Is there a part-time program that would allow you time to dedicate yourself to your education while continuing to work?

Guiding Philosophy and Frame of Reference

What is the school's frame of reference? What is its philosophy? How is its curriculum organized? Some curricula are organized developmentally across the life span; others are organized according to diagnosis, physical disabilities versus psychosocial dysfunction; still others are organized around occupation.

Degree Desired

Are you interested in pursuing a bachelor's or a master's degree? (Generally, an entry-level master's degree does not pay more initially, but opportunities for advancement later are greater.)

Are there related degrees you can obtain by taking only a few more classes that might advance your career even further? (For example, some programs can be arranged so that with only a few other classes you could also get your bachelor's degree in psychology.)

Prerequisites

Pay close attention to exactly what the prerequisites are. If you are a transfer student, will your courses transfer? Prerequisites may change from year to year. Different schools can have different prerequisites. At some schools, you may be able to apply to the OT program while still working on your prerequisites, but at others, the prerequisites must be completed prior to application. Know the school's policy so you do not waste its time or yours by applying when you are not truly qualified.

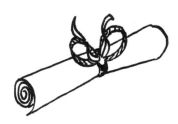

How Long Has This School Been Established?

There are many new programs being developed all the time. You may have a better chance for acceptance into a new program that is going through the accreditation process; however, you also take the chance that the school won't get its final accreditation. Remember, you must complete your educational program at an accredited school in order to take the national certification exam in the United States. Check other countries for their practice and examination requirements. Newer programs must provide all that AOTA requires, but they might not have as many clinical fieldwork experience options as more established schools have.

Does This School Offer Degrees in Closely Related Programs?

Many schools offer both an OT and a PT program. Do the various programs, faculty, and students have positive working relationships? Are there any shared classes? If you are not accepted into OT school, are there other closely related programs of interest to you? A college or university that offers other degrees related to medicine may have more clinical options available, such as a cadaver lab, and more resources in the campus library.

What Method Is Used for Matching Students to Fieldwork Sites and Is There an Option for a Third Rotation?

Who is offered first choice in making fieldwork selections? Does the fieldwork coordinator offer the opportunity for developing new placements in geographic areas where the program may not have placements established already? Is there an option

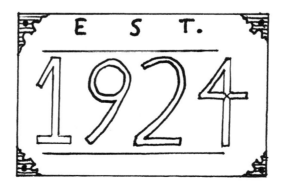

for a third rotation? Third rotations can be used for specialties if you already have a particular area of OT that you think you would really enjoy.

Are There Other OT Schools Nearby?

Is the local job market flooded with therapists? Would you be able to obtain an OT position in the area in which you wish to practice should you decide to stay in this geographic location? Are the fieldwork placement options limited because of the number of schools demanding placements from a limited number of hospitals and clinics?

How Much Clinical Experience Is Offered During the Program?

It is always a dilemma for schools to provide as much clinical experience as possible. Your Level I and Level II fieldwork placements are specifically designed to offer clinical exposure. However, how much lab time is offered within and outside of the classroom experience? Is there an on-site clinic?

When Does the OT Program Start and When Is the Application Due?

When is the application due? Can you have any outstanding prerequisites when you apply? (It is always recommended that you have your prerequisites taken care of before you start OT school because of the general intensity of the schooling.)

What Is the Class Size?

What is the teacher-to-student ratio? How many students per academic advisor are there? How many classes are there per year?

$$\boxed{9}$$

How to Apply to Occupational Therapy School

If you are at a college or university that offers an OT or OTA program, make sure that you have the following:

- Admission criteria
- Prerequisite courses
- Required volunteer or observation hours
- Required letters of reference
- Specialized testing that may be required, such as the Allied Health Professions Test, Graduate Record Exam, or Minnesota Multiphasic Personality Inventory
- Number of transfer hours allowable
- Specific departmental requirements, for example, specific documentation of criminal background check and community service hours

If you are at a school that does not offer an OT or OTA program but are planning to transfer to a school that does offer these programs, it is of the **utmost importance** that you make certain that the courses you have completed and are completing will transfer into the program to which you are applying. Make certain that you check with the registrar's office on the transferability of your past and current courses. Often schools have a transcript evaluator who can tell you before you enroll in the course whether or not it will transfer in and whether it meets a prerequisite course for OT applicants.

Schools have different requirements for prerequisite coursework and mandatory criteria for admission into their specific programs.

Step-by-Step Process of School Selection and Application

1. Review the listing of OT and OTA schools. Contact AOTA for this list at 800-SAY-AOTA.

2. Ponder the following questions:
   - What are your career goals?
   - What is the size of the institution? Some small colleges and universities may admit smaller class sizes for more personalized attention and learning. Therefore, you also need to think about your learning style.
   - Where would you like to be geographically? There are schools located throughout the United States and Puerto Rico as well as in other countries.
   - What are your financial resources? Most private learning institutions are more costly than are state institutions.
   - Would you consider applying to more than one school?
   - What are the unique properties of each program? Each accredited OT program meets standards established by the AOTA. Some schools, however, may have a certain specialty focus or therapeutic treatment philosophy. Read the mission statement for the college or university, as well as the OT departmental mission statement. Review the OT curriculum and the specific courses offered.
   - Are you ready to research different programs? It is of the utmost importance that you thoroughly explore what various educational institutions have to offer you.
3. Contact the OT and OTA programs in which you are interested. Remember that each college or university has different application processes, prerequisites, and deadlines for application. Allow ample time to obtain the information, complete an evaluation of the program, and proceed with the application process.
4. Inquire about the number of classes in the program on a yearly basis. Some schools admit just one class per year, whereas other schools may admit a new class each semester.
5. Inquire about the number of students admitted to the program on a yearly basis. Many programs admit a limited number of students. Although the university may have an enrollment of 26,000 students, the OT department may admit only 50 students each year.
6. Consider applying to more than one school. If you do, you will need to make certain that you have the application information from each school, as well as satisfy all prerequisites for each school.
7. Find out whether you must have completed all general education as well as prerequisite courses at the time of application. Many schools will not allow you to complete general education courses while you are in the OT program.
8. **Follow** the directions of the application process. Those processing your application at the various institutions are not going to call you to let you know if your application is incomplete. They typically have many more applicants than spaces to fill. Some schools may have more than 300 applicants for only 50 spots. It is your responsibility to see that your application is complete.
9. Keep in mind that admission requirements change, especially if you obtain information about various programs several years before you plan to actually

attend. You need to keep in close contact with the institution to ensure that you are charting your course properly by taking the correct courses required for admission as well as fulfilling any other admission criteria.

10. Ask the persons with whom you speak for their names when you contact institutions. This is important because one person may tell you one thing and someone else may tell you something very different. Therefore, it is also important to write down what information your contact gives you. It can be difficult to keep clear what different schools tell you when you are applying to a number of them. This advice applies for all departments within the institution, including housing, student life, financial aid, general education, or transfer student advisor, as well as the OT department.

11. Keep things in perspective. There is competition for admission to many programs. Constant worrying about whether or not you will be admitted is not productive. Do your very best in your current courses. OTs focus on keeping work, rest, and leisure in balance. Throughout your academic career, it is important to keep this concept in mind.

12. Turn in your application. Then it is just a matter of waiting, which can be extremely difficult. Have an alternative plan in place in case you are not accepted to OT school.

13. **If you were accepted:**
    - Make sure the institution has all the documentation it needs and that you have paid any fees associated with your admission to the program.
    - Call all your friends, family, and significant others and celebrate!

14. **If you were not accepted:**
    - Make an appointment to speak with an advisor in the department to discuss your application, strengths, weaknesses, and available options.
    - Consider retaking some courses in order to raise your GPA and reapply to the program or to other programs.
    - Consider applying to other schools that have different admission requirements.
    - Consider completing a bachelor of science degree in psychology or biology and applying to an entry-level master's program.
    - Participate in additional volunteer and observation experiences to expand your knowledge about the profession as well as to expand your people skills.
    - Consider other career choices in related fields.
    - Refer to the descriptions of related health-care professions as described in this text.

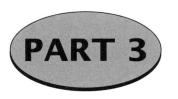

Observation Guidelines

(10)

Pretest for Observation Experience

Directions: Answer True or False in the blanks provided.

1. _____ OTs work mostly on finding people jobs.

2. _____ OT educational programs were first offered in the United States in 1918.

3. _____ OT is a career for females only.

4. _____ Crafts are used in OT to entertain patients.

5. _____ In the 1990s, the salary for an entry-level OT with a 4-year degree can range from $28,000 to $40,000+, depending on the geographic area in which the therapist practices.

6. _____ OTs are employed in hospitals, schools, community-based programs, industry, and large state-run institutions.

7. _____ OTAs have a 2-year college degree.

8. _____ OTs have to go to school for 6 years and have a master's degree to practice.

9. _____ The fastest-growing practice area in OT is working with elderly people.

10. _____ Since the 1980s, the number of OTs practicing in mental health has been on the decline.

11. _____ OTs often make upper-extremity splints for patients.

Professional Behavior Checklist

Professional behavior is important in OT. Before you begin a course of study leading to a degree in OT, it is wise to examine your strengths and weaknesses. Think about **your skills and abilities in an objective manner**. Complete the following professional behavior checklist on **yourself**. Being open to feedback from others is an important step in your professional development. Each individual has strengths and weaknesses. It is important to be able to examine areas you may need to change; therefore, it is important to your professional development that you be able to examine the feedback given by others and develop some realistic goals for improving your skills in those areas.

Characteristic	Excellent	Above Average	Average	Below Average	Poor
Interpersonal skills					
Reliability					
Initiative					
Integrity					
Educational curiosity					
Ability to accept criticism					
Flexibility					
Creativity					
Self-discipline					
Self-concept					

This form adapted in part from Occupational Therapy Department. St. Ambrose University, Davenport, IA 52803.

Questions for Thought and Reflection

Is there one area in which you believe you excel? How would that area be an advantage to you as an OT?

What is the area in which you rate yourself the lowest? What is a realistic and measurable goal that you could establish to improve yourself in this area?

Identify which area you believe is most important to your professional future as an OT. Why do you think this area would be essential to an OT?

Ask three people who know you well to complete the form on the following pages and give you feedback. These should be people with whom you have been acquainted a significant period of time who are able to rate your ability in all areas. Examples of individuals you might select to provide you with feedback include a coworker, a teacher or extracurricular advisor, or your past or present employer.

(12)

Professional Feedback Forms

Professional Feedback Form #1

Directions: The individual who has provided you with this form is interested in your feedback regarding his or her personal and professional abilities as they relate to an interest in a career in the profession of OT. For those not familiar with OT, a definition has been provided. Please review the definition and then complete the checklist and accompanying questions in an objective manner.

Definition of Occupational Therapy

Occupational Therapy is the use of purposeful activity or interventions to achieve functional outcomes. Achieving functional outcomes means to develop or restore the highest possible level of independence of an individual who is limited by a physical injury or illness, a dysfunctional condition, a cognitive impairment, a psychosocial dysfunction, a mental illness, a developmental or learning disability, or an adverse environmental condition.[1]

Characteristic	Excellent	Above Average	Average	Below Average	Poor
Interpersonal skills					
Reliability					
Initiative					
Integrity					
Educational curiosity					
Ability to accept criticism					
Flexibility					
Creativity					
Self-discipline					
Self-concept					

Which area(s) do you believe are strengths for this individual?

In which area(s) do you believe this individual could continue to grow and develop?

What are your suggestions for continued growth and development in these area(s)?

Knowing what you know about the profession of OT and the characteristics as identified above, do you believe this individual would be successful in pursuing an education in OT and, upon successful completion of such education, in practicing as an OT?

_____ Yes, without reservation.

_____ Yes, but I believe that the individual should closely consider the following:

_____ No; I believe from **what I know** about the profession of OT and what I know about this individual, this person would not be well suited to pursuing formal education and practicing in this area at this time.

Reference

1. American Occupational Therapy Association. (1993). Definition of occupational therapy practice for state regulation. *American Journal of Occupational Therapy, 47*(12), 1117.

Professional Feedback Form #2

Directions: The individual who has provided you with this form is interested in your feedback regarding his or her personal and professional abilities as they relate to an interest in a career in the profession of OT. For those not familiar with OT, a definition has been provided. Please review the definition and then complete the checklist and accompanying questions in an objective manner.

Definition of Occupational Therapy

Occupational Therapy is the use of purposeful activity or interventions to achieve functional outcomes. Achieving functional outcomes means to develop or restore the highest possible level of independence of an individual who is limited by a physical injury or illness, a dysfunctional condition, a cognitive impairment, a psychosocial dysfunction, a mental illness, a developmental or learning disability, or an adverse environmental condition.[1]

Characteristic	Excellent	Above Average	Average	Below Average	Poor
Interpersonal skills					
Reliability					
Initiative					
Integrity					
Educational curiosity					
Ability to accept criticism					
Flexibility					
Creativity					
Self-discipline					
Self-concept					

Which area(s) do you believe are strengths for this individual?

In which area(s) do you believe this individual could continue to grow and develop?

What are your suggestions for continued growth and development in these area(s)?

Knowing what you know about the profession of OT and the characteristics as identified above, do you believe this individual would be successful in pursuing an education in OT and, upon successful completion of such education, in practicing as an OT?

_____ Yes, without reservation.

_____ Yes, but I believe that the individual should closely consider the following:

_____ No; I believe from **what I know** about the profession of OT and what I know about this individual, this person would not be well suited to pursuing formal education and practicing in this area at this time.

Reference

1. American Occupational Therapy Association. (1993). Definition of occupational therapy practice for state regulation. *American Journal of Occupational Therapy, 47*(12), 1117.

Professional Feedback Form #3

Directions: The individual who has provided you with this form is interested in your feedback regarding his or her personal and professional abilities as they relate to an interest in a career in the profession of OT. For those not familiar with OT, a definition has been provided. Please review the definition and then complete the checklist and accompanying questions in an objective manner.

Definition of Occupational Therapy

Occupational Therapy is the use of purposeful activity or interventions to achieve functional outcomes. Achieving functional outcomes means to develop or restore the highest possible level of independence of an individual who is limited by a physical injury or illness, a dysfunctional condition, a cognitive impairment, a psychosocial dysfunction, a mental illness, a developmental or learning disability, or an adverse environmental condition.[1]

Characteristic	Excellent	Above Average	Average	Below Average	Poor
Interpersonal skills					
Reliability					
Initiative					
Integrity					
Educational curiosity					
Ability to accept criticism					
Flexibility					
Creativity					
Self-discipline					
Self-concept					

Which area(s) do you believe are strengths for this individual?

In which area(s) do you believe this individual could continue to grow and develop?

What are your suggestions for continued growth and development in these area(s)?

Knowing what you know about the profession of OT and the characteristics as identified above, do you believe this individual would be successful in pursuing an education in OT and, upon successful completion of such education, in practicing as an OT?

_____ Yes, without reservation.

_____ Yes, but I believe that the individual should closely consider the following:

_____ No; I believe from **what I know** about the profession of OT and what I know about this individual, this person would not be well suited to pursuing formal education and practicing in this area at this time.

Reference

1. American Occupational Therapy Association. (1993). Definition of occupational therapy practice for state regulation. *American Journal of Occupational Therapy, 47*(12), 1117.

Guidelines for Interaction with Patients

Confidentiality is of utmost importance. At many facilities an employee may be fired if he or she breaks the facility policy regarding confidentiality.

Review and sign the confidentiality statement per the facility or clinic policy.

- While at the facility, introduce yourself using your first name, and ask the patient's permission to observe his or her involvement in therapy. Do not become frustrated or angry if the patient refuses your request; it is his or her right to refuse.
- Do not discuss one patient's condition, progress, or treatment with another patient or anyone else except your supervisor.
- Be objective about the feedback that patients give you and statements they may make about other professionals working with them.

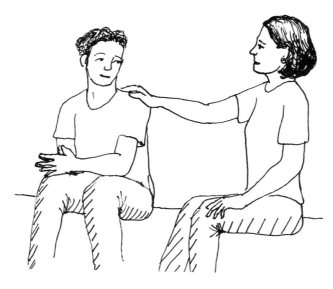

- Practice your empathetic listening skills; try to think what it would be like to be in the patient's shoes.
- Acknowledge the uniqueness of each patient, and address each patient equally during treatment sessions. Do not show favoritism between patients.
- Do not make promises to patients that you cannot fulfill.
- Many facilities have stringent policies concerning whether facility staff may accept gifts and so on from patients. Make sure to follow the facility policy.
- Ask the patient by which name you should address him or her, and ask for the correct pronunciation of the patient's name. Some elderly patients prefer to be addressed as Mr. or Mrs.; children may prefer a nickname.
- You are at the facility to observe therapy services and interact with patients. It is not your responsibility to give advice to the patients or their families.
- Make certain that you speak to the patient in a tone of voice that he or she can hear. This tone will vary from patient to patient.
- Do not talk about a patient with other professionals or with family members when around the patient, even if you think he or she is confused or cannot hear you.

(14)

Observation Assignment List

Directions: Here is a sample of an assignment list that you may go through prior to beginning your observation or volunteer experience. It may be customized to meet your learning needs as well as the needs of the facility or clinic where you are observing. This form is to serve strictly as a guideline.

1. Department orientation; obtain facility name tag.
2. Complete the student preassessment by the second session at the facility.
3. Read the department mission, philosophy, and operating procedure.
4. Complete the pre-OT quiz.
5. Read Chapter 2, "What Is Occupational Therapy?"
6. Read guidelines for patient confidentiality prior to orientation session.
7. Complete the "Adaptive Equipment Matching Activity" scavenger hunt (Chapter 29).
8. Complete at least four observation assignment sheets (see "Observation Worksheet for Practice Areas" in this book; you will need to photocopy it, since only one is provided here).
9. Assist the supervising therapist in demonstrating adaptive equipment.
10. Answer the departmental phone while in the office.
11. Assist with departmental photocopying.
12. Assist the therapist in engaging patients in therapeutic activities.
13. Assist the therapist in scheduling patients and transporting patients as assigned per facility policy.
14. Learn and demonstrate proper body mechanics when involved in clinic activities.
15. Assist the supervising therapist to lead groups per facility policy.
16. Complete a student log of patients observed (see "Observing Patients," Chapter 21).
17. Meet with supervisor on weekly basis or as needed; complete weekly report form.
18. Learn how to take blood pressure by practicing on an OT staff member.
19. Observe treatment of patients in PT and speech therapy.

20. Consistently assist in keeping the department neat and clean.
21. Complete "Career Opportunity Assignment" (Chapter 33).
22. Read "Current Working Conditions Within the Profession of Occupational Therapy" (Chapter 6).
23. Read an article in *OT Week* or *Advance for Occupational Therapists*, available in the department, and report to the staff on the contents of the article (5- to 10-minute talk). Ask the clinic supervisor for a relevant article from the *American Journal of Occupational Therapy* to see an example of clinical research in the field.
24. Read and ask questions about OT education: "How to Compare Occupational Therapy Schools" (Chapter 8) and "How to Apply to Occupational Therapy School" (Chapter 9).
25. Complete the posttest (Chapter 28) on the last day of your experience.
26. Sign a release of information (Chapter 25) and give it to your supervising therapist. Make certain you have any necessary documentation completed by your supervisor prior to your last day.
27. Learn a lot about OT and enjoy your experience!

Observation Orientation Documentation

Directions: This orientation form may be used as a guideline to ensure that the student doing the observing has been oriented to the topics that are essential within the facility or clinic. This may be accomplished by having the student observe other clinicians, complete readings independently during clinic time or prior to coming to the clinic, and ask questions in each area.

Procedure	Discussed/Demonstrated
Philosophy/mission	
Performance expectations	
Dress code	
Staffing patterns	
Departmental personnel	
Physical layout (refer to map)	
Disaster and fire procedures	
Safety procedures/universal precautions	
Infection control	
Patient transportation	
Material safety data sheets	
Observation experience schedule	
Phone/interdepartmental communication	
Patient evaluation	
ADLs	
CVA	
Hips/knees	
Group treatment	
Hands/splinting	
Pediatrics	
Home health	

Procedure	Discussed/Demonstrated
Therapeutic use of activities and crafts	
Patient/family/staff education	
Interaction guidelines with patients	

I understand the above information that was presented to me.

Student's Signature	Date	Supervisor's Signature	Date

(16)

Confidentiality Statement

The American Occupational Therapy Association Code of Ethics, Principle 2 states:

Occupational therapy personnel shall respect the rights of the recipients of their services (autonomy, privacy, confidentiality). Within this principle, the following areas are specifically addressed:

A. Occupational therapy personnel shall collaborate with service recipients or their surrogates in determining goals and priorities throughout the intervention process.

B. Occupational therapy personnel shall fully inform the service re-·cipients of the nature, risks and potential outcomes of any interventions.

C. Occupational therapy personnel shall obtain informed consent from subjects involved in research activities indicating they have been fully advised of the potential risks and outcomes.

D. Occupational therapy personnel shall respect the individual's right to refuse professional services or involvement in research or educational activities.

E. Occupational therapy personnel shall protect the confidential nature of information gained from educational, practice, research and investigational activities.[1]

It is important that you understand your responsibility regarding patient confidentiality. While you are at your observation experience, anything you hear or observe during patient contact and treatment is confidential information. This information may be discussed only with your supervisor or other clinicians with whom you are working. It is important to remember that this patient information should not be discussed with your family, your roommate, or other patients.

Most facilities have policies regarding patient confidentiality. Confidentiality is a serious professional responsibility. In many facilities, if a therapist breeches patient confidentiality, the therapist may be fired. Make sure that you understand the policy for confidentiality at the facility before you begin your observation or volunteer experience.

I have reviewed the following document and understand the importance of patient confidentiality.

Student's Signature	Date	Supervisor's Signature	Date

Reference

1. American Occupational Therapy Association. (1994). Occupational therapy code of ethics. *American Journal of Occupational Therapy, 48*(11), 1037–1038.

Preobservation Assessment

Directions: You should complete the following pages prior to beginning your observation experience. You should also share this information with your supervisors so they can understand your level of knowledge. These questions are designed to help you understand the different clinical practice areas in which OTs are employed and develop questions for your supervisors during your experience. It is assumed that you will have difficulty answering some of the questions if you have limited knowledge about the profession of OT. The questions are intended, however, to facilitate your thinking and help determine the areas where you need to increase your knowledge.

1. What were your previous clinical observation site(s)? What diagnoses did you observe?

2. What types of treatment have you assisted in or observed?

3. Have you had any special learning experiences, observations, opportunities, or volunteer experiences?

4. What level or type, or both, of supervision do you prefer? How do you learn best (e.g., through observation or verbal instruction or by assisting therapists)?

5. What are five important things to remember when meeting a new patient?

   1.

   2.

   3.

   4.

   5.

6. Do you have any medical conditions of which your supervisor should be aware (diabetes, seizure disorder, or weight restrictions for lifting)?

7. What are your objectives for this observation experience?

8. What personality attributes or characteristics do you have that will help you pursue your career as an OT or OTA?

9. Do you have any attributes or characteristics that you need to change to be successful in becoming an OT or OTA?

10. What interests you about OT?

11. What are some of the questions you would like to have answered regarding OT as a profession?

As you enter this experience, remember that supervision is a two-way street. Being a therapist means you need to constantly evaluate yourself and your performance. Your supervisors can assist you with this, but they cannot facilitate your learning if you are not willing to put forth the initiative. Remember to ask questions. Many people are afraid of asking a stupid question, but there is no such thing as a stupid question. Asking questions is an excellent method of facilitating your learning experience. Interaction within the experience is largely dependent on what you are willing to put into it. If you are committed and willing to put effort into the experience, chances are it will be a wonderful and rewarding experience for you.

(18)

Professional Terminology Exercise

Directions: For your observation experience to be meaningful, you need to understand certain professional terms that you will hear physicians, nurses, and therapists using. Prior to your observation experience you should look up the terms listed below in a dictionary or medical dictionary and familiarize yourself with them. Make note of any terms with which you are unfamiliar that you would like to discuss further with an OT. An excellent source for obtaining the definition of these terms is *Taber's Cyclopedic Medical Dictionary*. Most clinics have this text, or you could purchase one from a bookstore. This is a dictionary that you will refer to repeatedly throughout your professional career as an OT. After you have looked up these terms, you can ask your supervisor for more clarification or definition, if needed.

Activities of daily living

Activity

Adaptive equipment

Affect

Agonist

Aphasia

Apraxia

Aspiration

Ataxia

Balance

Beliefs

Blood pressure

Body image

Body scheme

Cock-up splint

Codependent

Cognition

Confusion

Crafts

Discharge planning

Dynamic splint

Dynamometer

Empathy

Endurance

Fine motor

Functional capacity evaluation

Goniometer

Grading (an activity)

Gross motor

Lethargy

Modalities

Occupation

Occupational performance

Orientation

Orthotic

Prehension

Proprioception

Prosthetic

Protective sensation

Purposeful activity

Range of motion

Seating/positioning

Sequencing

Standardized evaluations

Strength

Suicidal ideation

Time-out

Values

Visual-motor integration

(19)

Observation Worksheet for Practice Areas

Directions: Complete the following questions based on the practice area you are observing. Do not look up information in texts available within the department. You will not be graded on this assignment. The purpose of this assignment is to help your supervising therapist understand what you know about OT. Additionally, it is anticipated that you will not know the answers to some of these questions. These questions are meant to assist you in gaining an understanding about each of the practice areas listed.

Practice Area: Physical Disabilities

1. What behaviors and symptoms might you see when observing a patient who has sustained a stroke (cerebrovascular accident [CVA])?

2. What is the difference between quadriplegia and paraplegia?

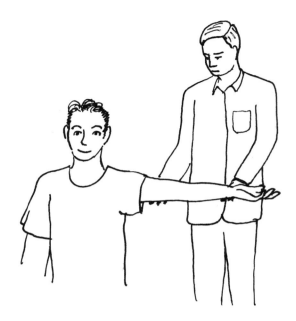

3. What are three activities a person who has had a total hip replacement (THR) might not be able to do?

    1.

    2.

    3.

4. What are five activities you could do with a patient who has visual-perceptual difficulty?

    1.

    2.

    3.

    4.

    5.

5. Can an individual with a physical disability, such as a spinal cord injury, live independently or is the individual typically placed in a structured living environment, such as a nursing home?

Therapists who work in a physical disabilities practice area work with patients who have a variety of diagnoses, including CVA, traumatic brain injury (TBI), THR, total knee replacement (TKN), multiple sclerosis (MS), spinal cord injury (SCI), and other conditions that may affect an individual's physical ability. Therapists who work in this area first evaluate patients to determine their level of functioning. After interpreting the information obtained from the evaluation, the therapist will work collaboratively with the patient to develop treatment goals that address the areas of dysfunction. Within the treatment setting the patient will be presented with therapeutic tasks to improve independence. Therapists may also teach patients how to use adaptive equipment that will help them complete tasks independently. OTs are holistic. In addition to addressing a patient's physical level of function, they examine the patient's psychosocial functioning. Patients may be seen in inpatient rehabilitation, outpatient rehabilitation, their own homes, or nursing homes.

Directions: Complete the following questions based on the practice area you are observing. Do not look up information in texts available within the department. You will not be graded on this assignment. The purpose of this assignment is to help your supervising therapist understand what you know about OT. Additionally, it is anticipated that you will not know the answers to some of these questions. These questions are meant to assist you in gaining an understanding about each of the practice areas listed.

Practice Area: Psychosocial

1. What behaviors and symptoms might you observe in a patient diagnosed with schizophrenia?

2. What behaviors and symptoms might you observe in a patient diagnosed with major depression?

3. What are three activities you could use to treat a patient with poor communication skills?

   1.

   2.

   3.

4. What are three activities you could use with a patient with poor coping skills?

1.

2.

3.

5. How are individuals diagnosed with a mental illness stigmatized by society?

Therapists who work in mental health work with patients who have a variety of diagnoses, from depression, schizophrenia, personality disorders, substance-abuse disorders, dementia, and anxiety disorders to other conditions that affect an individual's mental health and emotional well-being. Similar to therapists who practice in physical disabilities, therapists who practice in mental health areas will review the client's medical history, complete an evaluation, develop goals, and implement treatment. Within the treatment setting, the therapist involves patients in purposeful functional activities to address activities of daily living, stress management, development of coping skills, time management, communication, and task skills. Patients may be seen within inpatient mental health units, as part of partial hospitalization programs or community-based treatment, or at home.

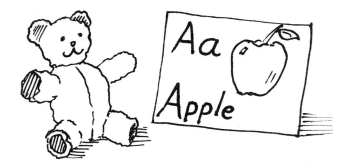

Directions: Complete the following questions based on the practice area you are observing. Do not look up information in texts available within the department. You will not be graded on this assignment. The purpose of this assignment is to help your supervising therapist understand what you know about OT. Additionally, it is anticipated that you will not know the answers to some of these questions. These questions are meant to assist you in gaining an understanding about each of the practice areas listed.

Practice Area: Pediatrics and School Systems

1. What behaviors and symptoms might you observe in a child diagnosed with cerebral palsy?

2. What behaviors and symptoms might you observe in a child diagnosed with attention deficit hyperactivity disorder?

3. What are five activities that a therapist would use for development of fine motor skills to address a child's difficulty with handwriting?

   1.

   2.

   3.

   4.

   5.

4. What would a therapist use to present activities to a child? (Hint: begins with the letter p.)

5. Are children with physical disabilities allowed in school classrooms with nondisabled children?

   Therapists who work in pediatrics might work in outpatient clinics, hospital-based settings on a pediatric unit or a neonatal intensive-care unit, in community-based early intervention programs, or within a preschool or school system. The therapist might work with children who have physical or emotional limitations that are interfering with their ability to complete activities independently at an appropriate age level. Children may have a diagnosis of cerebral palsy, attention deficit hyperactivity disorder, failure to thrive, learning disabilities, feeding or eating disorders, or developmental delay. Therapists who work in pediatrics must be patient and holistic in their approach to treatment. They work not only with the child, but also with the parents and siblings of that child. Since play is the primary occupation of the child, pediatric therapists use play as a primary method to build the child's developmental skills. The therapist may work within the classroom as a consultant, with a teacher, to help a child with difficulties function independently in classroom activities. The OT may initiate modifications, such as a larger grip on a pencil or placement of materials for independent access in the classroom.

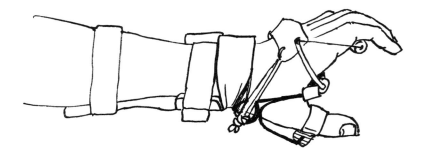

Directions: Complete the following questions based on the practice area you are observing. Do not look up information in texts available within the department. You will not be graded on this assignment. The purpose of this assignment is to help your supervising therapist understand what you know about OT. Additionally, it is anticipated that you will not know the answers to some of these questions. These questions are meant to assist you in gaining an understanding about each of the practice areas listed.

Practice Area: Work Hardening and Hand Therapy

1. What are the symptoms you might see when the therapist evaluates a patient with a hand fracture?

2. What are two common work-related injuries that an OT would see in a work-hardening setting?

    1.

    2.

3. What are five activities a therapist could use to improve upper-extremity strength?

    1.

    2.

    3.

    4.

    5.

4. Why is it important for a patient to use proper body mechanics consistently, especially when lifting?

5. What does "malingering" mean? Do you think that malingering could affect an individual's progress in therapy?

Therapists who work in work hardening and hand therapy work with patients who have a variety of diagnoses, including cumulative trauma disorder, back injuries, shoulder injuries, nerve impingement, tendon lacerations, and crush injuries. Therapists who work in this practice area evaluate patients and their overall level of function and may evaluate their job sites. Therapists may demonstrate proper body mechanics to patients as well as instruct them how to complete tasks in a safe manner. Hand therapists may use modalities such as ultrasound, fluid therapy, or paraffin as preparation for treatment. Patients with hand injuries may participate in range-of-motion exercises or be fitted for a splint custom made by the OT. Areas in which patients may be seen include outpatient treatment centers, physicians' offices, occupational health centers, or general hospitals.

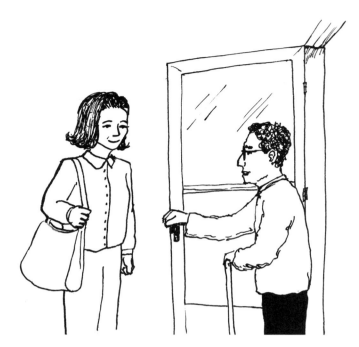

Directions: Complete the following questions based on the practice area you are observing. Do not look up information in texts available within the department. You will not be graded on this assignment. The purpose of this assignment is to help your supervising therapist understand what you know about OT. Additionally, it is anticipated that you will not know the answers to some of these questions. These questions are meant to assist you in gaining an understanding about each of the practice areas listed.

Practice Area: Geriatrics, Nursing Homes, and Home Health Care

1. What are three stereotypes that come to mind when considering the elderly population?

   1.

   2.

   3.

2. What are three problems that an elderly patient might have that would require OT treatment?

    1.

    2.

    3.

3. What are three activities you could use with elderly patients to improve their balance?

    1.

    2.

    3.

4. What are five activities to improve memory or problem solving, or both?

    1.

    2.

    3.

    4.

    5.

5. What are three benefits for the OT, as well as for the patient, when therapy is provided in the patient's home?

    1.

    2.

    3.

OTs working with a geriatric population may see patients who are diagnosed with Alzheimer's disease, arthritis, depression, CVA, THR, generalized weakness, chronic obstructive pulmonary disease, or Parkinson's disease. Therapists who work with geriatric patients evaluate the patient's level of independence, cognition, and safety. The treatment plan is designed to maximize independence and function. Generally, the therapist's goal is to return patients to their own homes. A therapist who performs home health-care services provides services to patients who may be unable to leave their homes. Therapists may recommend adaptive equipment, such as reachers, long-handled sponges, or shoe horns, to assist the patients in completing routine tasks with a greater level of independence.

Observing a Therapist

Reminder: Patient information is **confidential** and **must not** be shared with anyone except the supervising therapist.

It may be helpful to photocopy this sheet if you plan on observing several different therapists in several different settings.

Therapist's name _____

Date _____

Patient initials _____

Patient gender _____

Diagnosis _____

Date of onset of diagnosis _____

Date of admission _____

Physician's orders to OT and reason for OT referral:

Symptoms and behaviors observed during session:

Activities the therapist selected for the patient's involvement during the treatment session:

Are there any other activities you believe would be appropriate for this patient? Present your rationale why the activity would be appropriate and discuss it with your supervisor.

From your observation, identify one goal of the therapist and patient.

Was the therapist required to modify the activity in any way so the patient could engage in, participate in, or complete the activity? Was the activity purposeful and meaningful to the patient? How could you tell?

Describe any precautions taken by the therapist during the treatment session. List why it is so important to take these precautions.

How did the patient respond to the treatment session (active participation, cooperation with therapy, positive effect, improvement from last session)? What techniques did the therapist use to elicit the patient's cooperation (selecting an activity that was meaningful to the patient, talking with the patient about the progress being made, verbally encouraging the patient)?

Patient Observation Tracking Sheet

Facility name _____

Dates of observation _____

This information is confidential. Follow facility policy regarding confidential information.

Patient Initials	Diagnosis	Age	Comments: Specific Type of Assessment or Treatment Observed; Type of OT Services Provided

22

Adaptive Equipment Scavenger Hunt

Directions: Find the equipment in the rehabilitation department that best fits the descriptions provided here. Write the name of the equipment in the space provided. If this equipment is not available, do the Adaptive Equipment Matching Activity on page 115 instead.

A. _____ This item would be used to help you pull up your pants and get dressed.

B. _____ This item can be put around the plate to help you scoop food onto your fork or spoon.

C. _____ Someone using this item may have trouble walking without it.

D. _____ This item is used in the tub or shower for washing your back.

E. _____ If you could not stand up, this item would help hold you in place so that you could walk.

F. _____ A therapist would use this item to measure how far you could move your arms or legs, or both.

G. _____ If you could not bend over, you could use this item to put on your socks.

H. _____ If you could not stand in the shower or tub, this device could help you bathe or shower independently.

I. _____ This device holds your foot in the correct position for walking.

J. _____ This item is used to help you drink without spilling liquid.

K. _____ A therapist uses this device to assist a patient in moving from one place to another.

L. _____ This equipment is used to help you button your shirt and pants.

M. _____ If you could not grasp something in your hand, this device could help you hold onto it.

N. _____ This device is used to reach things on the floor without bending over or to reach things on a high shelf.

O. _____ This item is used to prevent sores from developing on your bottom.

P. _____ This device is helpful if you want to eat ice cream and cannot move your wrist much.

(23)

Time Management and Scheduling

Directions: You may use this schedule to develop and individualize your schedule during your observation experience. Effective time-management skills are very important for practicing clinicians. It is appropriate for you to develop these skills at this time. On this schedule, document where you will be throughout the day. For example, at 8:00 a.m. you will be observing Laura working on ADLs with a patient in his room; at 8:30 you are to watch Dee fabricate a splint in the clinic; and at 9:30 Christine will be leading a group in the mental health unit.

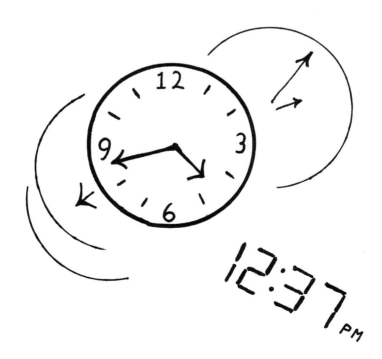

Hour	Sunday	Monday	Tuesday	Wednesday	Thursday	Friday	Saturday
6:00 a.m.							
6:30							
7:00							
7:30							
8:00							
8:30							
9:00							
9:30							
10:00							
10:30							
11:00							
11:30							
12:00 p.m.							
12:30							

Hour	Sunday	Monday	Tuesday	Wednesday	Thursday	Friday	Saturday
1:00							
1:30							
2:00							
2:30							
3:00							
3:30							
4:00							
4:30							
5:00							
5:30							
6:00							
6:30							
7:00							
7:30							
8:00							

24

Observer and Supervisor Weekly Report Form

Date _____

Supervising therapist over the last week _____

What specific questions or issues would you like to discuss?

Are the expectations regarding your observation or volunteer experience clear to you?

How are you benefiting from this experience?

What type and degree of feedback have you received from your supervisor?

What are you learning about OT through your observations?

What strengths have you noticed in yourself during the observation period?

In what areas would it be important to improve as you pursue a career in OT?

Release of
Information Form

Note: This release of information form is provided as a sample. It is wise to check its legality in your geographic area.

I, _____, hereby authorize and request therapists

at _____ (name of facility) to release information regarding my participation in an observation experience at the aforementioned facility.

Release to:

_____

_____

_____

    I understand that I have the right to revoke this consent at any time. I understand that I have the right to inspect and copy the information to be disclosed. I understand that refusing to sign this form will prevent information regarding my observation from being released to prospective schools.

    By signing this form, I release and hold blameless the aforementioned facility, its employees, agents, and members of the medical staff from any and all liability that may arise due to authorized disclosure of student or volunteer information from all or a portion of my experience or record.

Consent will expire _____ (not to exceed 2 years)

Signature _____   Date _____

Witness _____   Date _____

(26)

Supervisor's Evaluation of Observation Experience

Name of Observer _____

Name of Facility _____

Facility Address _____

Name of Supervisor _____

Dates of Observation Experience _____

Hours of Observation Completed _____

Directions: Based on your observation of the student during this experience, please rate the student in the following areas using the rating scale provided.

1 = Poor (fails to meet standards)
2 = Fair (meets requirement but requires cuing or prompting)
3 = Good (adequately meets requirement)
4 = Very good (meets requirement; quality is evident and appropriate)
5 = Excellent (exceptional; quality evident in meeting or exceeding requirements)
N/A = Not applicable (not observed at this setting)

Please comment on areas in which a score lower than 3 is given.

Criteria	1	2	3	4	5	Comments
Professional Characteristics General appearance is appropriate to the setting						
Is punctual and reliable						
Demonstrates positive work habits						
Is self-disciplined						
Flexibility						
Educational Curiosity Initiates questions and clarifies areas of uncertainty						
Demonstrates a willingness to learn						
Shows an interest in the facility, observation experience, and clients						
Interpersonal Skills Demonstrates an ability to relate to others and work with individuals of varied backgrounds, ages, and functional limitations						
Effective written communication						
Effective oral communication						
Demonstrates ethical behavior						

Adapted from Level I fieldwork rating form. St. Ambrose University, Davenport, IA 52803.

What do you believe are this student's strengths?

What suggestions do you have for the student's continued professional growth and development?

Please comment on any other area of student performance not addressed on this evaluation.

Supervisor's Signature _____ Date _____

Student's Signature _____ Date _____

Observer's Evaluation of Experience

Name of supervisor(s) _____

Dates of observation experience _____

1. Was your orientation sufficient?

2. Was the observation experience structured to meet your identified needs and goals?

3. How did your experience help you learn more about OT and treatment of patients with different abilities?

4. Was supervision provided as needed?

5. Was constructive feedback provided appropriately and in a timely manner?

6. Were the assignments in this manual helpful?

7. How did this learning environment challenge you?

8. What additional learning experiences would you have liked to have?

9. What was most helpful to you during this experience?

10. What was least helpful to you during this experience?

11. What overall comments or suggestions would you offer regarding this experience?

_____   _____
Student's signature   Supervisor's signature

28

Posttest of
Observation Experience

Directions: Answer True or False in the blanks provided.

1. _____ OTs use adaptive equipment to help patients gain independence after an injury or illness.

2. _____ ADL stands for activities of daily living and includes bathing, dressing, and feeding.

3. _____ OTs do not believe in using purposeful activities, which may include crafts, cooking, games, and so on, for treatment.

4. _____ OTs work only in hospitals.

5. _____ OTs may complete a bachelor of science degree or an entry-level master's degree, whereas OTAs complete an associate degree.

6. _____ Very few OTs practice with the elderly.

7. _____ Both males and females can pursue a career as an OT.

8. _____ OTs mostly work to find people jobs in the community after an injury or illness.

9. _____ An OT and a nurse would complete the same tasks in their daily jobs.

10. _____ Being an OT would be a very boring job.

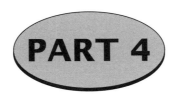

Other Learning Activities

Adaptive Equipment Matching Activity

Directions: If you do not have the equipment available to do the Adaptive Equipment Scavenger Hunt on page 97, do this activity instead. Place in the space provided the number of the picture that **best** matches the description of the equipment pictured.

A. _____ This item would be used to help you pull up your pants and get dressed.

B. _____ This item can be put around the plate to help you scoop food onto your fork or spoon.

C. _____ Someone using this item may have trouble walking without it.

D. _____ This item is used in the tub or shower for washing your back.

E. _____ If you could not stand up, this item would help hold you in place so that you could walk.

F. _____ A therapist would use this item to measure how far you could move your arms or legs, or both.

G. _____ If you could not bend over, you could use this item to put on your socks.

H. _____ If you could not stand in the shower or tub, this device could help you bathe or shower independently.

I. _____ This device holds your foot in the correct position for walking.

J. _____ This item is used to help you drink without spilling liquid.

K. _____ A therapist uses this device to assist a patient in moving from one place to another.

L. _____ This equipment is used to help you button your shirt and pants.

M. _____ If you could not grasp something in your hand, this device could help you hold onto it.

N. _____ This device is used to reach things on the floor without bending over or to reach things on a high shelf.

O. _____ This item is used to prevent sores from developing on your bottom.

P. _____ This device is helpful if you want to eat ice cream and cannot move your wrist much.

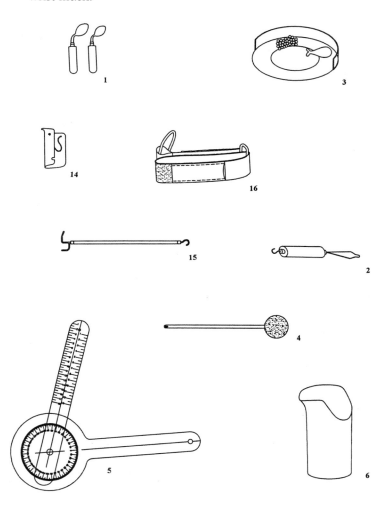

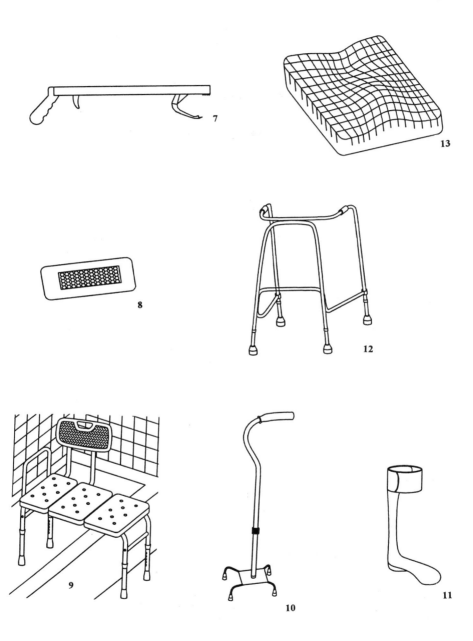

7

13

8

12

9

10

11

30

Disability Experience Exercise

There are a number of methods to simulate having a disability. In simulation, how-ever, you only experience what it would be like to have a disability for a limited amount of time. These experiences are intended to facilitate your thinking about what an individual who has a disability must address on a daily basis.

Upon completion of one or all of these six scenarios, you may choose to spend an entire day with people who have a disability in order to continue developing your understanding of disability and function. If you participate in this activity, as the in-dividuals go through their day, make note of the activities in which they participate; how they perform the activities, either independently or with assistance; and the com-munication they share with you. It is important not only to observe individuals in their daily routines, but also to listen to what they comment on while completing the routine.

Another suggestion is to keep a journal about all the activities you engage in for 1 day and 1 week. Then, analyze the activities you engage in on a regular basis. Would you be able to complete these activities independently if you had one of the functional limitations described here?

Directions: Select one or all of the following six scenarios and complete the activity as directed. After you complete the activity, answer the accompanying questions. This will help you understand how an individual with a disability would approach completion of routine tasks. The activity will also help you understand how an OT might grade an activity. When OTs do grade an activity, they find methods or use equipment to simplify a task so an individual might perform without assistance or with as little assistance as possible. (In treatment sessions, a therapist may make an activity more difficult to challenge the patient.[1]) At the end of the sixth scenario (see Chapter 31), a brief description of how a therapist would assess and treat an individual who is experiencing this type of limitation is presented. Therapists base their assessment and treatment of clients on specific theoretical principles.

Experience #1: Paralysis of Dominant Upper Extremity

When you are getting dressed in the morning and completing your morning routine, do not use your dominant hand and arm. You must complete all activities in your routine: getting undressed, selecting your clothes, getting dressed, brushing your hair, brushing your teeth, preparing your breakfast, eating your breakfast, cleaning up after your breakfast, and washing any dishes you have.

Questions for Thought and Reflection

What was the most difficult part of completing your morning routine?

How did completing your morning routine without the use of your dominant arm affect the amount of time it took you to complete these usual activities?

Were you able to complete all of the activities independently or did you need assistance from someone?

If you requested assistance, how did you feel about this person's providing the assistance you requested?

What would you have done (or what did you do) if there had been no one available to help you to complete the task with which you were having difficulty? Would you have skipped that activity for today? Would you have asked someone at work to help you? How would your self-esteem be affected if you required assistance for completion of this activity on a routine basis?

How would you feel if you were unable to use your dominant arm to complete your morning routine again?

What would have to happen for you to successfully adjust to this change in your independence and abilities?

What other difficulties do you feel you might encounter if, in addition to not being able to use your dominant arm, you were also confined to a wheelchair?

Is there any adaptive equipment that would be appropriate for use by a person who has limited movement in both the upper and the lower extremities?

Experience #2: Visual Impairment

Take a pair of sunglasses and wrap plastic wrap over them. Then get out the materials you need to make a peanut butter and jelly sandwich. You must keep the glasses on the entire time you make the sandwich. Make sure to get something from your refrigerator to drink, because peanut butter makes you thirsty. Pick up your dishes, wash them, and put them away.

Questions for Thought and Reflection

What was the most difficult part of completing this activity with your vision impaired?

Do you think you would be able to prepare a meal, including meat, potatoes, salad, vegetable, and dessert? How long do you think it would take you to accomplish this task? Do you feel you could safely prepare this meal with your vision impaired?

Were you able to prepare the sandwich and wash the dishes without assistance? If you needed assistance, how did you feel about requesting it?

If your vision was impaired like this all of the time, what are some other activities with which you might encounter difficulties? Do you feel you would have trouble driving a vehicle, caring for a small child, or working on needlework?

How would you feel if you were dependent on someone else to prepare all of your meals, and you had no input on the type or quantity of food that was prepared for you?

What would you do if, in addition to your vision being impaired, your ability to sequence steps of a task were impaired? What if, while completing this activity, you were only able to recall how to do two steps in the sequence and then were unable to recall how to complete the activity, an activity you had successfully completed many times before?

Experience #3: Sensory Impairment

Gather eight cotton balls and tape them to your fingertips with masking tape. Do not put them on your thumbs. Go to your computer keyboard or typewriter and try to type a letter to your best friend. The letter must consist of at least one paragraph.

Questions for Thought and Reflection

How many typing errors did you make the first time you tried to type? How long did it take you to type the paragraph? If you are typically a skilled typist, did this frustrate you?

What would you do if you were not able to communicate orally, the computer was your only means of communication, but your sensation was impaired? How would this limitation affect your communication?

What other activities would be difficult to complete with tactile sensation in your fingers limited?

Is there any activity you feel would be unsafe without your finger sensation? How could you compensate for your limited sensation during these activities?

How would you perform your normal routine activities of daily living if your hearing were impaired as well as your tactile sensation?

Is there any adaptive equipment appropriate for an individual experiencing sensory loss that would assist in the completion of daily tasks?

Experience #4: Auditory Hallucinations Often Experienced in Diagnosis of Schizophrenia

Put on a portable radio or tape player. Put the volume at a level low enough that you can hear it but not the normal volume at which you listen. Find someone with whom you would like to have a conversation. While wearing headphones, try to have a conversation lasting at least 10 minutes with this person. Next, make a list of items you need to purchase from the grocery store or make a list of things you need to accomplish over the next week.

Questions for Thought and Reflection

Were you able to have a conversation while wearing headphones? Were you able to stay on topic, follow the discussion, and contribute appropriate information?

Were you able to concentrate on the task of making a grocery list without the music distracting you? Many people listen to music while completing other activities, but if the music were replaced by people's voices and you could hardly hear what they were saying, do you feel it would be more distracting?

What are some activities you would have difficulty completing if you were constantly hearing music or voices in your head and you did not know whether or not the music and/or voices were real?

Are there any activities you feel would be unsafe if you were hearing voices? With which activities would you need to ask for assistance?

How would completing your daily routine be difficult if, in addition to hearing voices, you felt so anxious that you could not sit still and constantly worried about everything? How would this affect you?

Experience #5: Depression

In private, imagine a time in your life when you experienced extreme stress (e.g., break up with a partner, death of someone close to you, moving away from home) or felt your life was out of control. As a result of this stress, you feel depressed and somewhat anxious.

Questions for Thought and Reflection

How would these stressors affect your ability to complete your activities of daily living? Do you feel your motivation to get up, shower, dress, and go to your job would be impaired? If so, how?

Because of your depression, your appetite has decreased, and you are only eating one small meal a day. How would this affect your ability to function effectively?

What is your normal reaction pattern when other people come to you with their problems or difficulties if you are already feeling overwhelmed yourself?

Are there any activities you feel you would have difficulty completing because of your depression?

In addition to feeling depressed, you were just diagnosed with diabetes. What impact would this have upon your work, self-care, and leisure activities?

You decided to seek help for your depression and were put on medication by a psychiatrist. One of the side effects of the medication is dry mouth. Your job requires you to be on the phone for 7 of the 8 hours you work each day. How would you cope?

Your friends and family try to cheer you but do not understand the diagnosis of depression. They say you need to just "pick yourself up by the bootstraps." How would this statement make you feel?

Experience #6: Cognitive Limitation

Purchase a boxed brownie mix. Read the instructions on the back of the box and, with a black marker, cross off every third step in the directions. Now, prepare the brownie mix according to the modified directions. For example, if the mix says add egg, water, and oil, the oil is the third step and you would leave out the oil. Bake the brownies.

If you have made brownies before, you have experience in completing this task. Do not make brownies for this activity; rather, complete an activity you have never completed before without any written or verbal instructions.

Questions for Thought and Reflection

How did the brownies turn out? Did you skip the step that required you to stir the mix for 3 minutes? Did you skip the step that said bake until toothpick inserted comes out clean? What did your brownies taste like? Were they fit for human consumption?

What activities might be dangerous for you to participate in if you could not successfully sequence the steps of a task or your attention span was impaired? Do you feel that cooking and driving are activities that you could perform safely?

To whom would you look for support if, according to your OT, you are unable to perform activities such as cooking or driving safely? Would you try to perform these activities without regard to the recommendations of the therapist? How would you feel if you were unable to drive and had to depend on another person for transportation all of the time?

Do you have any ideas of how you could structure the brownie-preparation task so that none of the steps would be omitted by a person who is experiencing cognitive limitations?

Reference

1. Keilhofner, G. (1997). *Conceptual foundations of occupational therapy* (2nd ed.). Philadelphia, PA: F.A. Davis.

(31)

Discussion of Occupational Therapy Assessment and Treatment of Simulated Disabilities

Disability #1: Paralysis of the Upper Extremity

Assessment

A therapist assesses the following areas in an individual who is experiencing paralysis of the upper extremity:
Endurance
Amount of movement in both upper extremities
Strength of both upper extremities
Fine-motor coordination
Sensation
Level of independence in activities of work, self-care, and leisure
Patient's level of motivation to participate in therapy

While assessing the patient's overall function, the therapist will be screening for any cognitive deficits. This screening can be accomplished by assessing the client's ability to follow verbal directions given by the therapist. If the client exhibits confusion, this impairment would be noted.

Treatment

There are many conceptual practice models that can be used to address this type of disability, some more adept at addressing the dysfunction than others. Kielhofner[1] points out, however, that the method of intervention must not only match the identified limitations, such as motion, strength, and endurance, but also address the underlying causes of these limitations.

Activities that are purposeful and functional and have meaning to the patient and that will increase the patient's range of motion, thereby increasing independence in work, self-care, and leisure activities, are selected by the therapist. Depending on the therapist's theoretical model and the patient's goals, the therapist may choose to maximize the weakened upper extremity functioning and then work on maximizing the patient's independence with activities of daily living. The therapist may also have the patient work on adapted activities, such as one-handed dressing, while working on strengthening the upper extremity.

Disability #2: Visual Impairment

Assessment

Safety awareness
Frustration tolerance
Level of independence in activities of work, self-care, and leisure
Patient's level of motivation to participate in therapy
General upper extremity functioning: motion, strength, and sensation
Cognitive deficits (problem solving, memory, sequencing, comprehension)

Treatment

The therapist will select activities that are functional for the patient to interact with the environment and to facilitate independence. It is also helpful to adapt the environment to maximize safety and independence.

Disability #3: Sensory Impairment

Assessment

Sensory examination of both upper extremities: assessing the ability to sense hot or
   cold, sharp or dull pain
General upper extremity functioning: motion and strength
Level of independence in activities of work, self-care, and leisure
Patient's level of motivation to participate in therapy
Cognitive deficits (problem solving, memory, sequencing, etc.)

Treatment

The therapist will work on adaptation of the environment to compensate for sensory losses and instruct the individual to access and use adaptive equipment in the activities of work, self-care, and leisure to compensate for limited sensation. The individual will be educated about skin care and methods to request assistance or delegate tasks that may be difficult to complete and what tasks might put them at risk for injury.

Disability #4: Auditory Hallucinations

Assessment

Willingness to participate in therapy; signs of paranoia, tension, or guardedness, which will provide the therapist with the initial task of developing a therapeutic rapport before any further assessment
Determination of the individual's reality orientation
Assurance that the individual is in a safe environment
Determination of what areas (work, self-care, rest, leisure) are being affected by the individual's symptoms of schizophrenia
Examination of the level of social functioning (Often individuals who are experiencing auditory hallucinations are quite paranoid and guarded, and their social functioning may be affected as a result.)

Treatment

Individuals who are experiencing auditory hallucinations benefit more from involvement in tasks in which the activity is the focus. These individuals demonstrate difficulty with groups primarily focused on discussion and social interaction.[2] Appropriate activities for these individuals address patient deficits such as self-care activities and structured leisure activities, as appropriate. These activities should be structured.

Disability #5: Depression

Assessment

Current coping and stress-management abilities
Motivation
Problem-solving and decision-making abilities
Performance areas that might be affected by the depression, such as ability to complete grooming tasks, socialization, home management, and educational, work, and leisure activities
Time-management skills
Interests and activities the individual is pursuing on a regular basis need to be addressed

Treatment

The therapist works to address deficit areas during the assessment phase. This work might include an activity that motivates the individual as well as provides a sense of reward or fulfillment. The therapist addresses the individual's stress level and current coping abilities and collaborates with the individual to establish goals for behavioral change to improve or increase the individual's role performance abilities (ability to complete work, self-care, education, and leisure tasks independently).

Disability #6: Cognitive Limitation

Assessment

Independence in activities of daily living
Attention span
Problem solving
Decision making
Comprehension
Sequencing
Safety in performance of everyday tasks

Treatment

The therapist develops compensatory strategies for cognitive deficits that became apparent during the assessment and rearranges or adapts the environment to facilitate independence in the client.

References

1. Kielhofner, G. (1997). *Conceptual foundations of occupational therapy* (2nd ed.). Philadelphia, PA: F.A. Davis.
2. Posthuma, B. (1989). *Small groups in therapy settings: Process and leadership*. Boston, MA: Little Brown.

(32)

Observation Experiences Without an OT

Observation Experiences Without an Occupational Therapist: #1

To increase your knowledge about the profession of OT, you may choose to complete some self-study and then explore areas where OTs may be employed. For example, in your community, there may be one or more nursing homes. Geriatric practice is an ever-growing and changing area of practice within OT. You may spend some time observing at a nursing home where there are no OTs employed to develop observation and communication skills and interact with a variety of individuals. It would be best if you could observe at a facility where there is an OT. Some regions of the United States and Canada have a limited number of OTs, however. Engaging in this type of activity will help you develop professional behavior and skills. Within the nursing home setting you could possibly:

Observe or assist clients during mealtimes
Observe or assist during structured activities with an activity director
Observe or assist certified nursing assistants as they help clients complete activities of daily living such as bathing, grooming, and dressing

After spending time in this setting, consider the following questions:

What areas of difficulty did you observe as clients performed their daily activities or occupations?

Are there any changes that could be made to improve their independence and potentially increase their quality of life?

With your current level of understanding of the profession of OT, what do you think the role of an OT would be within this type of setting?

If there were an OT employed within this setting, what are some questions you would like to ask? (These may be helpful questions that you ask another OT you meet in the future.)

Observation Experiences Without an Occupational Therapist: #2

Consider what services are available within your community. Are any of the following services available: adult day care, adult group home, respite care, homeless shelter, battered women's shelter, community mental health day treatment, or senior citizen congregate meal site?

Locate an agency that offers one of the listed services or some other type of service to individuals diagnosed with a disability.

Spend time with the clients at that agency as a volunteer. To increase your knowledge about the various services provided to clients with disabilities, answer the following questions:

Describe the environment in which the services are provided to clients.

Does this environment facilitate client independence?

Describe the needs of the clients.

What types of services are provided?

What professionals provide these services?

Do you think there is a place for an OT within this agency?

With what you know about OT at this time, what do you think the role of an OT would be within this setting?

How do the services at this agency increase the quality of life of the clients served? What do you think would happen if these services were not provided?

Observation Experiences Without an Occupational Therapist: # 3

An additional experience you may choose to expand your knowledge and understanding of disability is to spend time with an individual diagnosed with a disability. During this experience, document the activities of this person while you are together. If you could spend an entire day together, from the time the person arises until the time he or she retires for the evening, it would be very beneficial. Remember that it is of utmost importance that you are respectful of the wishes of the person. If this individual states that you may spend 3 hours, respect that limit and do not press for more time. You do not want the individual to feel as if he or she is under a microscope during your time together. During your experience with this person, observe his or her activities. Then, consider the following:

What are this person's life roles (caregiver, home maintainer, friend, worker, student, etc.)?

In what way do you feel the individual's disability affects these roles?

What tasks did the person perform differently from how you usually do them? Did the person complete these tasks differently as a result of the disability or is this his or her standard method of task completion?

What modifications of or adaptations to the environment did you observe during the time you spent together that helped this person be independent?

What activities do you feel this person may have difficulty completing independently because of the disability?

How would you describe this person's quality of life?

Is there anything that you feel would improve this person's quality of life?

Knowing what you do about the profession of OT, do you think that an OT has ever provided treatment for a person with this disability? What do you think the role of an OT might be in treating an individual diagnosed with this type of disability?

33

Career Opportunity Assignment

Two publications that advertise positions for OTs are *Advance for Occupational Therapists* and *OT Week.* There may be copies of these publications in the OT department where you are observing. Select several different issues of these publications and look through each. In the back of each publication you will find job advertisements from hospitals and clinics that want to hire OTs.

Read through the listings and find five job opportunities that interest you. You may base your decision on area of practice; would you like to work with children (pediatrics), with the elderly (geriatrics), in hand therapy, in mental health, or in the schools? You could also base your decision on where you want to live, for example, the Midwest, the East Coast, and so on. Another factor to consider is the salary offered. This should not be your only consideration, but it is something you should consider.

Briefly list the name of the facility and the information mentioned in the advertisement that attracted you to the position. Review this information with your supervisors and listen to the feedback they may provide.

The purpose of this activity is to give you an idea of all the opportunities and areas where an OT may be employed. Additionally, this activity can help you identify areas where you might complete clinical fieldwork experience. When you are in OT school, you will have to complete a minimum of 6 months of Level II fieldwork for an OT and 16 weeks for an OTA.

If you are interested in applying to an entry-level master's degree program, it would be beneficial for you to obtain a copy of and review several articles from the *American Journal of Occupational Therapy* (AJOT). This is the primary professional journal for OTs in the United States and will provide you with some idea of the clinical research that is being done within the profession. The *Canadian Journal of Occupational Therapy* (CJOT) is another excellent source of information about research being completed in the profession.

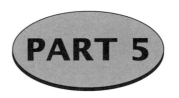

Conclusion

(34)

Goodbye and Good Luck!

The authors of this book want to offer you a sincere good luck wish! This book started out as a very small notebook in a small OT department. It was, and still is, based on our empathy; we can recall very easily what it was like applying to OT school and being an OT student. We love our profession as OTs and hope that future students continue to improve themselves and the profession overall. We appreciate everyone's help and interest with this book and look forward to your comments.

Please forward comments to:

Laura Anderson, OTR
and Christine Malaski, MS, OTR
c/o Lynn Borders Caldwell
F.A. Davis Company
1915 Arch Street
Philadelphia, PA 19103
Email: lbc@fadavis.com

or

Post your question to "Ask the Author" at the
F.A. Davis Company web site: www.fadavis.com

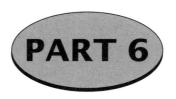

Appendices

Additional Resources

For more information regarding the profession of OT contact

American Occupational Therapy Association (AOTA)
P.O. Box 31220
Bethesda, MD 20824-1220
301-652-7711
http://www.aota.org

The AOTA has numerous publications and videos available to increase your knowledge about OT. For information more specific to the U.S. region in which you are interested, request a listing of state OT associations from AOTA.

A list of accredited OT and OTA programs is published annually in the November/December issue of the *American Journal of Occupational Therapy*. You may request a list of programs from AOTA, as well.

If you are interested in obtaining information about OT in Canada, contact

Canadian Association of Occupational Therapists (CAOT)
Carelton Technology & Training Centre
Suite 3400
1125 Colonel By Dr.
Ottawa, ON K1S 5R1
800-434-CAOT
http://www.caot.ca

If you are interested in obtaining information about OT in Australia, contact

Australian Association of Occupational Therapists, Inc. (AAOT)
6 Spring St.
Melbourne, VIC 3065
Australia
61-3-9416-1021
Fax 61-3-9416-1421

If you are interested in OT in other areas of the world, contact

World Federation of Occupational Therapy (WFOT) President
Ms. Barbara Tydsley
Saxon Lodge
6 Huyton Church Rd.
Liverpool
L365SJ
United Kingdom
Fax 44-51-794-5719

APPENDIX

Answers for Quizzes

Pretest

1. False
2. True
3. False
4. False
5. True

6. True
7. True
8. False
9. True
10. True
11. True

Adaptive Equipment Matching Activity

A. 15
B. 3
C. 10
D. 4
E. 12
F. 5
G. 14
H. 9

I. 11
J. 6
K. 8
L. 2
M. 16
N. 7
O. 13
P. 1

Posttest

1. True
2. True
3. True
4. False
5. True

6. False
7. True
8. False
9. False
10. False

151

APPENDIX

C

High School Courses Helpful in Preparing for an Occupational Therapy Education

College course preparation is required. The following courses in high school may be helpful to prepare you for your college career:

- Biology, Chemistry, and Physics
- English and any writing courses (4 years)
- History or Social Studies
- Languages
- Mathematics (3 years)
- Computer Science
- Psychology or Sociology (or both)

Other opportunities to take advantage of if they are offered at your high school may include:

- Work-study programs that would put you in a health-care or human-services setting (These provide you with on-site experience and help you to learn good work habits early.)
- Art, music, and theater extracurricular activities to help you expand your creativity
- Sports activities to help you maintain or improve your wellness and learn about your muscles and body
- Writing opportunities (yearbook, school paper, etc.)
- Leadership activities
- Travel or cultural experiences
- Sewing, foods, industrial arts courses (Many of the activities learned in these classes involve activities of daily living or activities you may use in treatment with patients.)[1]

Even high school is not too early to work on balancing your life among work, play, leisure, and self-care activities. Getting involved in extracurricular activities (as long as they are balanced with your studies) is wonderful and provides fun learning experiences.

Reference

1. Abbott, M., Franciscus, M.L., & Weeks, Z.R. (1988). *Opportunities in occupational therapy careers.* Lincolnwood, IL: NTC Publishing Group.

Index

Adaptive equipment, 97–99, 115–117
Auditory hallucinations, 125–126, 133

Case manager, 26–27
Certified nurse assistant, 27–28
Certified occupational therapy assistant (COTA), 10, 43–44
Cognitive limitation(s), 129–130, 134
Confidentiality, patient, 64, 70–71
COTA (certified occupational therapy assistant), 10, 47

Depression, 127–128, 133–134
Dietitian, 22–24
Disability experience exercise, 118–130

Education and professional training, 10, 30, 45–52, 152–153

Geriatrics, 90–92

Hallucinations, 125–126, 133
Hand therapy, 88–90
Health professions related to OT, 13–28, 39
High school, course(s) of study, 152–153
Home health care, 90–92

Job outlook, 38, 141
Journals, professional OT, 141, 149

Licensure and examination procedures, 30

Nurse(s), 24–25, 27
Nursing homes, 90–92

Observation experience(s)
 assignment checklist, 66–67
 confidentiality statement, 70–71
 disability experience exercises, 118–130

general information, 3–8
for geriatrics, nursing homes, and home health care, 90–92
observer's evaluation of, 107–110
observer's weekly report form, 103
orientation documentation, 68–69
patient interactions, guidelines for, 64–65
patient observation tracking sheet, 96
for pediatrics and school systems, 86–88
for physical disabilities, 81–83
posttest of, 111
preobservation assessment, 72–74
pretest for, 55
professional behavior checklist, 56–57
professional feedback forms, 58–63
professional terminology exercise, 75–80
for psychosocial disabilities, 84–85
release of information form, 103
supervisor's evaluation of, 104–106
supervisor's weekly report form, 102
time management and scheduling, 99–101
with a therapist, 93–95
without a therapist, 135–140
for work hardening and hand therapy, 88–90
worksheets for, 81–92
Occupational therapist (OTR)
 certified assistant (COTA), 10, 43–44
 daily tasks performed by, 10–11
 education and professional training, 10, 30, 45–52, 152–153
 employment options, 11, 39
 licensure and examination procedures, 30
 observing a. See Observation experience(s)
 practice areas, 31–32, 81–92
 roles/responsibilities of, 32–33, 43–44
 work setting for, 10
Occupational therapy (OT)
 adaptive equipment, 97–99, 115–117
 as a career, 34–37, 141, 149–150
 defined, 9, 29
 geriatrics, nursing homes, and home health care, 90–92
 health professions related to, 13–28, 39
 history of, 9
 job outlook, 38, 141
 observations in. See Observation experience(s)
 in pediatrics and school systems, 86–87
 philosophical assumptions in, 11

155